Dominique Sakoilsky started her journey with birt
when she had her first child in 1988, and has worked in the arena of
birth ever since. Her own birth experiences include a 5-week premature
birth in hospital, an unattended home birth (he was in a hurry) and
a home water birth.

　　　　Her passion for birth led her to train over twenty-five years ago
as an Active Birth teacher with Janet Balaskas and she worked at the
Active Birth Centre in London for ten years. She then also trained and
worked as a Relate Counsellor, a Family Counsellor, a Scaravelli-inspired
yoga teacher and a Craniosacral Therapist, working as part of a team at
The Bristol Centre for Craniosacral Therapy. Dominique has spent the
last three years studying with Karlton Terry in perinatal education.
Dominique has also been training doulas and childbirth educators
both privately and within the NHS for over fifteen years, and in 2007
co-founded Relaxed Birth and Parenting (relaxedbirthandparenting.
com) which is a training and educational company. She has a busy
practice in Bristol where she runs antenatal workshops, parenting and
yoga classes, counselling and cranial sessions, and continues to learn
with joy and inspiration from the families and individuals she works
with. She intends this book to bring forward a sense of freedom and
joy, whilst finding a way to engage with the challenges of birth.

Seven Secrets
of a Joyful Birth

Dominique Sakoilsky

Foreword by Janet Balaskas
Edited by Jessica Adams
Images by Karni Keogh
Front cover photography Leticia Valverdes

SilverWood

Published in paperback by SilverWood Books 2012
Reprinted 2013, 2014, 2017
www.silverwoodbooks.co.uk

ISBN 978-1-78132-689-3 (paperback)
ISBN 978-1-78132-007-5 (ebook)

British Library Cataloguing in Publication Data
A CIP catalogue record for this book is available from the British Library

Set in Myriad Pro by SilverWood Books
Printed on paper sourced responsibly

Contents

Foreword
by Janet Balaskas

This book is a true blessing for pregnant women, fathers to be and unborn babies. As you go through the incredible life change of starting a family, you have at your side, a very wise teacher to guide you, help you to understand, to inform and accompany you through this journey of a lifetime.

There are many good books and birth preparation 'methods' available these days, which offer invaluable practical guidance, including my own. What makes this book stand apart, is that it truly addresses the inner transformation that takes place in you as your baby develops in the womb, as you go through the adventure of birth together and beyond. It honours the unfolding from within that occurs as you grow emotionally from woman to mother, man to father, couple to parents and sometimes single parent. As your family is forming and taking its unique shape.

This book invites you to work through 'seven secrets'. When I first read the title I thought perhaps it would be a bit of a formula. However as I read the text I began to rejoice in the process. Even for me, now becoming a grandmother for the fifth time, it had relevance.

Today it is well known that what happens in the womb and around the time of birth has great relevance for our future – it's like a blueprint that establishes our emotional and physical health for years to come. Naturally we want to help our babies to grow and develop to their full potential. We want to help them through the birth process without trauma, we want to nurture them and respond to their messages and their needs appropriately. This book invites you to become more aware of yourself or yourselves first, so that you can be fully present for your baby as you share this adventure together.

In my view this is the number one responsibility of relating as an adult and of parenting. It is also the key to an easier, pleasureable and more relaxed pregnancy and birth. In the event that the unexpected happens along the way you will be empowered to make decisions and choices from your own inner wisdom and not from fear – your own or anyone else's.

I welcome this book wholeheartedly. It addresses the life process of having a baby in an imaginative and creative way. It fills a big gap in the current literature and in the care of pregnant mothers.

Our bodies and our hearts are designed for joyful birthing and parenting. As you hold this book in your hands, know that you have chosen a marvellous guidebook for the journey.

Dominique has a voice that leads you to your own truth. Clear, non-prescriptive, honest writing that comes straight from the heart and connects us with ourselves, our vulnerabilities, strengths and instincts.

It is also a book that is not afraid to honour the sacred, the spiritual aspects of living through this journey. I find this incredibly comforting. To know that we are held and guided in life's journey by forces greater than ourselves. It's not all up to us. We can let go and let life and birth unfold in all their majesty.

Enjoy this wonderful book, work with it and trust the process. It has the power to inspire you to grow in self awareness and to transform yourself, at a time that could not be more appropriate.

Janet Balaskas
June 2011

SEVEN SECRETS OF A JOYFUL BIRTH

Introduction

Working with pregnant women for over 20 years now has continued to surprise and inform me as to quite how much birth touches us in all areas of our life. The mechanics, or physiology, of birth are such a small part of the process. Birth touches our deepest fears and our deepest hopes. It challenges us about how we surrender to trust, how we go into the unknown and how we are able to let go in such monumental proportions, in such ways that we may never thought possible. Birth calls forth relationship issues, sexuality issues and self-acceptance in our journey to meet and welcome another being. There is a being separate from us yet inside us, affected by the choices we make and the pregnant body it inhabits.

The *Seven Secrets of a Joyful Birth* is not a book offering prescriptive ways about 'how to' birth. It is not a book written by any kind of expert or authority. It does not seek to give you advice. Rather it is an invitation to explore your journey through pregnancy, birth and early parenting, highlighting those areas which may be useful for you to give attention to – those areas that are individual and personal to each of us.

I never know what a woman may need in order to feel as relaxed and confident as possible as she approaches her birthing. I am always delighted to walk that journey of exploration with her, offering her tools along the way but knowing that ultimately she is the expert about herself and her birthing. I truly believe that, when women are able to make their own authentic choices around birth, then they will be able to ask for the support they need, while staying connected to themselves and to those around them.

A dear colleague of mine is always reminding me that we 'birth how we live'. So, I say, let's live with a degree of self-awareness at this time. Knowing yourself, what is touched by this experience and why, means that you will be free to respond to the birth without carrying a huge backpack of unacknowledged and undealt with 'stuff'. We don't have to fix this stuff, stuff which is simply the accumulation of life experience. Instead, the intention of this book is to bring into your awareness anything that may be making the journey one that is heavier than it needs to be.

Sometimes it is by attending to just the tiniest of things that we can breath more easily and step more lightly forwards. Often we are pulled down and pulled back by something that simply needs acknowledgement. Women appear to benefit from looking at a variety of different aspects of their lives, from firming up the boundaries in relationships with significant family members, to acknowledging past miscarriage, fear of the unknown or feeling good enough for the job. We can never assume that we know what needs our attention without giving it some thought. There is always a place at birth for the random, the unexpected, and this book may be a way of bringing attention to the random or those bits that we hadn't quite realised needed our attention.

One of the women I had the pleasure of interviewing using the *Seven Secrets of a Joyful Birth* questionnaire told me that she felt she was approaching birth 'uncoated'. English wasn't her first language, and when we looked at what this meant for her she revealed that she was actually wondering whether or not it was OK to approach birth feeling so vulnerable. When we begin to understand the hormones that are needed in birth, which this book will help to do, then we will be able to see that softening into a vulnerable, uncoated state is ideal.

We often confuse being vulnerable with feeling weak and unprepared. But when it comes to birth, preparing with knowledge and tools and then being able to let go to and allow the 'I'm not sure how this will be for me' to be there is the magic that's needed to help us birth most freely. It allows us to bring all of us to the table, not hiding some part away ourselves or feeling the need to be in denial. When we feel only part of us is welcome at our birth, then we use energy that we may need for birthing trying to control that part of ourselves. What I hope to bring forward is the idea that there is not one bit of ourselves that we need to hide. There is not one bit of ourselves that is not welcome on this journey. Our humanness in all its glorious forms can be acknowledged as being part of the miracle that is birth. We need not waste energy hiding stuff away that we don't deem relevant or useful. This is where the 7 words system comes in, the psychological toolkit upon which this book is based and which gives rise to the Seven Secrets of a Joyful Birth. It is a system that serves to bring forward the more hidden aspects of our psyche. Parts that if left hidden may disrupt the flow of our birthing journey. The 7 words should be held lightly, for it simply offers a point of exploration, nothing more, nothing less. It may help us to uncover increasing ways to lean into this experience and to find the balance between commitment and clear intention, and surrender and trust.

If there is a lack of peace within us, the 7 words may just help us to understand why, and what we may do to bring a depth of understanding to the situation. It is both profound and pragmatic in application. Nothing is too small or too big for it to help. The 7 words of authentic communication was created by a wise man and Sufi called James Burgess, who offers the idea that all human interaction can be concentrated in 7 words, or 7 states of being: No, Hello, Thank you, Goodbye, Please, Sorry and Yes.

James suggests that if we are clear about what we are thinking, then we are clear in our communication and clear action will follow. In this book I have attempted to devise a way that may bring clear thought, clear communication and clear action to the arena of birth. I want us to have fun on our journey to meet our loved one, while not denying the intensity of the experience for everyone involved, including our baby.

So, use this book with a sense of willingness, have fun, and maybe you will learn something new about yourself. Maybe the way you prepare for your birth will not be as you saw it, but will take some unexpected turn that enables you to birth in a way that is truly yours. Find your own way, nobody else's. This is your experience to be shared with your child, your partner and whoever else you choose to have there. Make it a cooperative venture between all of you. Use the Seven Secrets questionnaire (see p15) to explore what needs attention, so that enough of you is taken care of to a level which allows you to really let go.

While it will require courage, finding the inner confidence to make this journey so authentically yours will bring much joy. Following your own voice and seeking your own guidance is not much cherished at these times. There are endless books and classes telling you how to birth, how to parent, how to be. But this book challenges and supports you to find your own way, while offering areas to reflect on, tools that may serve you and questions that will help you to discover what you bring to birth.

There is something both intimate and profound about sharing with those around us from a place of inner confidence. This has certainly been my experience when exploring the Seven Secrets of a Joyful Birth with the women and families who I have been so privileged to join with in their birth preparation. So, let's let the coats that we hide in drop away, and allow ourselves to relax and to enjoy the journey.

Seven Secrets Questionnaire

This questionnaire is designed to help you identify which secret of a joyful birth will be most helpful for you to focus on in your birth and early parenting preparation. Find a quiet place and give yourself time away from any distractions. The questionnaire is divided into seven keywords, each representing one of the Seven Secrets of a Joyful Birth. Approach the questionnaire secret by secret, answering the questions in each section as honestly as possible as you go.

Score each answer on a scale of 1 to 10, where 1 is a definitive No and 10 is a definitive Yes. It can be helpful to ask a close friend to read each question out aloud to you and for them to jot down your score for each question. Do not spend too long thinking about your answer to each question, go with the first response that comes into your mind, this will probably be the most truthful. Once you have completed the questionnaire, follow the instructions that follow.

NO
Boundaries ~ Identity ~ Choice ~ Truth

Are you preventing people from interfering with your birth preparation?	
Do you acknowledge the existence of another being growing?	
Do you have a clear sense of what you want for your birth?	
Are you being honest with yourself?	
TOTAL	

HELLO
Attention ~ Openness ~ Exchange ~ Communion

Are you giving your pregnancy the attention it merits?	
Are you open to new ideas about birthing?	
Are you giving and receiving enough about your birthing?	
Are you connecting deeply with your baby?	
TOTAL	

THANK YOU
Appreciation ~ Valuing ~ Giving ~ Heart ~ Essence

Are you appreciating your pregnancy?	
Are you taking steps to value your pregnancy?	
Are you giving loving attention?	
Do you follow your heart in your birthing?	
TOTAL	

GOODBYE
Realisation ~ Decision ~ Completion ~ Moving On

Do you acknowledge you have entered a new time in your life?	
Are you making clear decisions to support this change?	
Do you follow through on your decisions?	
Is it easy for you to let go of the past?	
TOTAL	

PLEASE
Vision ~ Intention ~ Cooperation ~ Prayer

Do you have a clear vision for the arrival of your children?	
Do your actions support this vision?	
Are you receiving the support you need?	
Is this a spiritual experience for you?	
TOTAL	

SORRY
Responsibility ~ Remorse ~ Repair ~ Release

Are you taking responsibility for the baby?	
Can you allow yourself to be less than perfect?	
Have you faced your fears?	
In preparing for the birth are you releasing old resentments?	
TOTAL	

YES
Permission ~ Acceptance ~ Agreement ~ Surrender

If necessary will you permit appropriate intervention?	
Can you accept your birth may not go according to plan?	
Are you ready to say yes to your baby with enthusiasm?	
Are you ready to surrender to trust and go with the flow?	
TOTAL	

Now you have completed the questionnaire, total up your score for each section. The section with the lowest score will highlight which secret may be most helpful for you to focus on in your birth preparation. Read this chapter of the book first and then look at any other chapters that you are drawn to, or read all remaining chapters.

If you score evenly for each section, return to the questionnaire and do it again. Are you being completely honest in all your answers? The sections in which you score the highest indicate those areas in which you are strongest and, at the present time, you will find most comfortable to work with in your birth preparation.

You can return to the questionnaire at anytime during your pregnancy since every time you revisit it you may learn something new about yourself and where you are in this journey.

Throughout this book you will see case studies which focus on women who have completed the Seven Secrets Questionnaire. There have been some times when I have done the questionnaire with women right before birth. All the women in these case studies had put a lot of energy and commitment into preparing for birth so they seemed to score high in all areas. There wasn't too much for us to explore on these occasions but I think they benefitted from feeling ready and seeing it in this way, and so approached birth with confidence which seemed to bear out in their birthing.

1 No

Finding Your Truth

The first secret of a joyful birth is: Learn how to say 'No'. No is often regarded as a negative word. We may be afraid to say No in case people don't like us, because it seems uncompassionate or because we believe we are closing the door on other opportunities – or a combination of all these things. However, saying No is one of the most powerful and empowering things we can do for ourselves and others. Relaxing into our No allows us to be clear about who we are, it defines our identity, making it easier for us to relate to others, and it brings with it the freedom of committing to those things we do want to welcome into our life. If we have found it difficult in the past, then pregnancy and birth are the perfect opportunity for us to practise saying No. By doing so we gain confidence in ourselves, which naturally carries through into parenting, with innumerable benefits for us, our babies and our relationships.

No

When we start with the word No, we can get clear about what we don't want in our life. This kind of clarity enables us to unearth what we do want as the journey through pregnancy and on towards birth and parenting unfolds. Ideally, preparation for birth and parenting begins before conception; yet many of us come to it much further along than this. But, where are we? We're here. Now. So, we can let go of the past and concentrate on what is important – we have arrived at this point, it has brought about a new awareness and something has shifted within us. We describe birth and parenting as a journey since the most important thing is always where we are in the present moment. Sure, what we do now affects what happens later but the goal is not to reach an end, the journey is always changing and evolving, which is what makes it so captivating. With this attitude we can appreciate wherever we are for what it is – whether that's the moment we realise we've conceived, in the midst of the sensations of a contraction or making eye contact with our baby for the first time.

The Culture Of Birth

Whether we aware of it or not, throughout our whole lives we are fed

20

messages about what is normal for a woman in labour. The ideas, images and stories that circulate in society, in the media, and among our family and friends all inform our ideas about birth. During pregnancy, however, we are likely to become acutely aware of the culture of birth to which we have been exposed. In the West this is predominantly one of fear and medical emergency, yet every woman will have her own unique idea about what birth entails and for every horror story there is one of joy, spirituality and personal growth.

To begin exploring our beliefs around birth, we might start with some gentle enquiry, laying aside any judgment as we do so. We could ask: What is normal in birth? Is it hard? Easy? Painful? Blissful? Something women have to endure? Or, is it birth an experience they might enjoy and celebrate? Is it a purely physiological process? Or does it have important spiritual aspects too? Do we identify with the dominant Western medicalised culture of birth? Or are we associated with a sub-culture, such as natural, active, hynobirthing or yoga birth?

Engaging in this kind of questioning allows the patterns of our beliefs to emerge. As we become aware of our beliefs, our stories and ideas, around birth, we can then start to make a more active choice around which beliefs we wish to reject. By saying No to those beliefs which won't serve us well in birth and parenting, we are a step closer towards what is truthful for us in our birth. In this way, when spoken honestly, No is a wonderful opportunity for us to connect more deeply with our sense of Self.

Being Free To Say No

No often carries with many negative connotations and there can often be profound resistance to accepting the need for a clear state of No in our lives. Yet, being free to say No means we are able to present a very authentic 'Yes' (more about Yes in chapter two). When our No is sincere, open and not bound up with pleasing others, we can be as happy to say No as we can be to say Yes. By saying No, we can assert our territory – an important part of the nesting instinct in pregnancy – and be more aware of who we choose to spend time with, who we include in our circle of friends and where we seek support. On the flip side, if we do not have a clear No, we may let people and thoughts into our life that do not support us. Consequently, we may feel bombarded with information, overwhelmed by choice, or weighed down by demands. Saying No is a choice and, though it is not always an easy thing to do, failing to exercise such a choice may leave us feeling drained, exhausted, weak and unprepared to face the warrior challenges brought forth by birth and parenting.

From Ourselves To Others

When we discover we are pregnant, it is us and us alone that must stand in realisation of our pregnant state. Of course, our partner, baby and significant others may be deeply involved in this process too, but first we need to come to terms with the news and make sense of it ourselves. If we can give ourselves the space to be clear about how it feels to be pregnant, then it will be easier to come together as a family. By allowing ourselves this space, we are not separating from our partner or baby, simply recognising the value in being there for ourselves first so that we can then be more present for others. By getting clear about our pregnancy, we pave the way for clearer communication with our partner. Yet, it's not just women who may need time to get use to the reality of being pregnant. Fathers will certainly need time to reflect on the news too. If both partners are honoured with a reflective period, which is not selfish even though it may feel that way, things will be much easier further down the line.

Once this space has been made, we need to remain open to a whole range of possible responses and emotions. Just as we can let go of the idea of No being a negative word, we can let go of the idea of positive emotions being 'good' and negative emotions being 'bad'. Pregnancy is often a time of profound ambivalence. For instance, when a woman who has planned her pregnancy finds out she is pregnant, it may bring up unexpected and contradictory feelings that might appear strange to an outsider. Conversely, a woman who thought she wasn't ready for children yet, may have an unplanned pregnancy and surprise herself by responding with quick acceptance and joy at the news. All emotions are valid and deserve recognition. It is when emotions are pushed beneath that they become a problem; when released, they leave us with more energy and freedom to respond to life.

The Body Knows No

Pregnancy is full of surprises. As well as experiencing unexpected emotions which make up our truth about what it is to be pregnant, we may also become aware of our body in a new way. The body is an exceptional truth-teller and may frequently be our best guide in this life-changing journey – paying attention to this is vital at this time. The pregnant body often says No in a way that we are unused to prior to pregnancy. If we have pelvic pain or backache, we could ask: What is my body trying to tell me here? It may be that it is quite clearly saying No to fast-living and asserting its need to slow down. Begin by noticing when it feels relaxed and well, and when it feels tired and stressed. Many of us live in a constant state of low-level stress so we may only get glimpses of it at first but, if we start to cultivate awareness, we can gradually become familiar with how we feel when we are relaxed. With this awareness, we can begin to say No to situations, friends, relatives or work commitments that have a negative affect on the body, which is a profound way of nurturing the pregnant self.

Strengthening Your No

Saying No is not always easy. It is often something that takes practice before it becomes more natural. Begin by thinking about the following questions: Do you find it difficult to say No? Do you often feel imposed upon? Do you say Yes too quickly and then feel pressure to do things you don't really want to? When you do say No, do you often go back on your word?

If you answered Yes to any of these questions, then you may need to strengthen your No. The first thing you can do is start by allowing yourself some time to consider your responses before you make a commitment to a demand at work or a social invitation. Instead of saying Yes or No straight way, you could instead say: 'That sounds good, but I need to check a few things first. Can I get back to you as soon as I have done this?' You then have time to consider a truthful answer.

Some people are able to say No with ease and grace. But not all of us are blessed with this ability. If, for example, you have grown up in a family where it wasn't OK for kids to say No, or if you have developed people-pleasing tendencies, then giving yourself this time to accept or reject an invitation enables you to connect with your true self before you say yes or no.

If you find it difficult to know what the answer is straight away and there is a sense of confusion between what your head and heart are telling you, then first try and get a body-feeling of what it would be like to say yes or no. Visualise yourself in each scenario and feel how it responds. Imagine and feel what it would be like to say Yes, and then imagine and feel what it would be like to say no. As you do so, let go of any notions of should or shouldn't or perceptions of what other people might think. If you feel a sense of relief and are energised and relaxed, then this is probably the right answer. If you feel a sense of fatigue, heaviness and tension, then this is probably the wrong answer.

Next, take a day to notice practice connecting with your No more deeply. Carry a notebook around with you and jot down how many times in one day you are called upon to say No, and how honestly you do that. You may be quite surprised by what you have recorded at the end of the day.

As you begin to feel more practised in your No, you can start to turn your attention to your pregnancy and birth choices. Start with simple choices like whether you really want to go out tonight after work or whether you actually need to go home and rest. From here, you will soon build the confidence to consider bigger decisions, such as who you would like in the birthing room and what kind of things will help you relax in labour.

Keywords

No is the quickest and clearest way to get in touch with what is truthful for us in this moment. It offers a very real and honest place for us to return to – a place where we can examine what is significant for us at this time, free from the opinions and agendas of others. No allows us to be true to ourselves, making less room for resentment and more room for joy as we approach birth. We can now begin to refine our understanding of No with four keywords: boundaries, identity, choice and truth.

Boundaries

Boundaries are about cultivating self-respect. They are an expression of what is acceptable for us in our life, and what is not, and they enable us to communicate our wishes to others. When we set good boundaries in relationship, for instance, we can respond to its challenges from a more relaxed place. As we nurture good boundaries, we learn to bring our needs into relationship in a clear and balanced way and, by establishing strong foundations in other key relationships during pregnancy, we may then more easily begin to accommodate the needs of our baby.

Boundaries are of central importance to a baby's life in the womb. It is now understood in the field of birth psychology that babies receive all kinds of information from the mother via the placenta and umbilical cord, as well as telepathically, with different hormones relating to various emotional states. Pre- and peri-natal psychologists

– researchers specialising in babies' experiences in utero, which they regard as first nine month's of a baby's life and immediately before and after birth – suggest that an important knowing for a baby is that the mother establishes appropriates boundaries and lets them know that the emotional states, if upsetting, are the mother's and the mother's alone. Therefore, babies need not take on any of mum's experience as their own.

As well as giving baby an easier ride, it also liberates mum from such self-critical thoughts as: 'I shouldn't be feeling so sad/distressed/ stressed/angry?' Establishing boundaries, by simply talking and explaining what's going on in our life to baby, either in our head or out loud, allows us to be authentic about our feelings. It protects baby by letting them know that they don't need to worry about our present emotional state, however strong that may be. Denying emotions is not healthy or helpful. Part of being human is feeling emotion, and this is something baby needs to understand too. So, we can begin practising No and establishing good boundaries while a baby is in utero by communicating with them in the following ways:

- By taking ownership of the strong emotions. For instance, saying to baby: 'This is my anger, and I take full responsibility for it'.
- By explaining to baby that our emotional state has nothing to do with them and that we are sorry for any strong emotions and hormonal responses that they may be feeling as a result.
- By reminding baby that they are safe, loved and wanted. Mum may be expressing strong feelings, but she can take care of this situation herself.

This kind of communication with babies may challenge mainstream beliefs about the sentient knowing of babies in the womb – when does a baby become a being that is able to feel and perceive things about the world around them? Is this at the moment of conception? Before conception? At 12 weeks? Or once it is born? Yet, if we tune into our heart and instinct, we may be surprised to discover that we already have some sense of our baby's personality and a feeling of communicating with them on a soul level that we had not previously been able to express.

Boundaries have an important function for mother too. By exploring our boundaries, we create the opportunity to connect with our unique sense of Self, and to learn to accept and celebrate our individuality. It is about making a stand for who we are and what we believe in. This brings both strength and maturity. Boundaries help us establish feelings of safety and protection, which are necessary for a healthy pregnancy and birth.

When our boundaries are strong in a subtle way – that is, we are able to relax into them because we understand they are an essential foundation for a healthy life – we find that, not only do other people challenge us less but, when we do say No, we no longer have to do it in a forceful or aggressive way, or feel defensive about our choices. It is a great advantage to labour with a clear, relaxed sense of boundaries, so that we do take any combative energy into the birth itself – birth is not the place to be a battle axe! Clarity around boundaries enables us to soften into the process and makes it easier for us to communicate openly with birth attendants.

Moreover, the ability to distinguish the boundaries between what is outside and what is inside is vital information for labour. During labour, the woman's focus needs to stay deep inside herself, withdrawn from the external world. We need to be able to close ourselves off from the distractions of the external world, so that we can work with the powerful forces within. Allowing the outside to inhibit the inside is one of the main ways of hampering the birth process.

In physiological terms, women use the old, animal and instinctive part of their brain to birth – which thrives in a warm, softly-lit environment and an atmosphere of trust, reassurance, security and privacy. By contrast, the newer 'thinking' part of our brain, or neocortex, which likes questions, conversation and bright lights, can get in the way of birth. I hear the following words from women so often they have almost become a cliché: 'As long as I could go into my 'zone', I could cope with the pain and it was fine… But, as soon as I felt pulled out of my zone or became distracted, the pain became a lot worse.'

So, we can ask: Where are we in terms of boundaries? Do we have a definite sense of what is OK for us, and what is not? Are we able to stick by this, even amid the push-me-pull-you tides of social pressure? During pregnancy we will probably be privy to everyone else's opinion about our birth choices. But, if we are clear about which choices support our truth, then we can avoid getting swept away by others' beliefs. After all, our truth isn't the 'truth', it's simply a personal truth that feels right for us – and it is important because it speaks of our individuality, our unique spirit.

Identity

The second key word of No is Identity. If we think about our life and the things that make up our identity, we can see that we associate ourselves with certain feelings, thoughts, group of friends, activities, career choices, possessions, with a particular nationality or a certain religion or spiritual practice. What we value in life, and the personal characteristics we value in ourselves and other people, also contribute to our sense of identity.

These many different aspects of ourselves reflect something about us, they are the outer expression of who we are – and at the same time they tell us something about our identity too. Throughout our life we are subject to a wide range of inputs from our family of origin, schooling, friends and community. We then integrate these influences and make them our own. This is what makes us so special, an individual expression of life force. Within the same family, for instance, children may have very similar upbringings but process them in quite dissimilar ways. As a result they may appear quite unlike one another, even though they share some family characteristics.

During pregnancy, women often compare themselves to others, their style of maternity clothing, their bumps, the way in which they are coping with symptoms and how they are making their way through their choices around birth. It is easy to put pressure on ourselves to be a certain way, which can lead to self-critical thoughts such as: 'I should be feeling this by now... I shouldn't be feeling like that... I should be happy... more connected to my baby... more prepared for birth…' Internally, we might be going over any number of 'shoulds' and 'shouldn'ts'.

Rather than experiencing pregnancy as a period of intense self-criticism, however, we could instead embrace it as an opportunity to revise our current identity, to look at whether the choices we are making reflect our identity, and to orientate ourselves towards the woman and mother we want to be. After all, identity is not as fixed as it is sometimes thought to be. On the contrary, it has great fluidity. We are constantly changing and refining our sense of who we are as we shift and change from one moment to the next, filtering the world and our experiences into a set of values and behaviours as we move through our life.

By bringing awareness to this constant process of receiving information and experience, and then integrating it into what already resides within us, we gradually become clearer about the behaviours and choices that follow. So, we should question what it means for us, as an individual, to be pregnant. This is likely to be quite different to what it means for the woman sitting next to us in the antenatal clinic or our pregnant neighbour with three older children next door.

For instance, the way in which we conceived our baby will inform our identity as a pregnant women – we may have got pregnant unexpectedly and to much surprise, or we may have been through three miscarriages and IVF treatment before being able to sustain a pregnancy. Every unique conception scenario will have its own challenges and feelings attached to it, and every individual will process these in a different way. Identity is all about those big questions: Who am I? What am I? But we needn't be intimidated by these questions. We can simply start by noticing how we interact with the world, what language we use to communicate with others and who we allow into our personal space. These are all invaluable ways in which we can start to learn something about our identity.

Nurturing Identity

Ask yourself the following questions so that you can begin to get a sense of who you are and what you bring to this pregnancy, to this birth and to parenting this child. Answer as honestly as you can.

- What is it about you as a person that will serve this child well in their life?
- What qualities do you bring from your life and family experiences that will be of great benefit to your child?
- What don't you want to pass onto this child? What experiences of parenting have you had that you think would be unhelpful for this child?

Choice

In order to make strong choices, first it is necessary to rule out what we don't want. Through a process of elimination we can then define or get closer to knowing what we do want. So, choice is the next step in working with the state of No. Having established good boundaries and gained a clearer understanding of our identity, we can then express our identity through the choices we make.

When confronted with the numerous choices there are to consider around birth, it is completely normal to feel overwhelmed. If this is our first baby, everything may be completely new. But even if we have had two or more children, we may feel like we're starting over again since there may be things we want to do differently this time – and birth is never the same twice. Initially, we could go anywhere and everywhere with our ideas about what we want for our birth. However, it is in the choosing that we find freedom. Options keep the mind busy and distracted but, to make choices that are right for us, we need to drop into a deeper place within ourselves. Through active choice comes commitment, and with that comes an enlivened sense of personal power. This is what is truly helpful in preparing for birth. Nevertheless, we need to be clear that we are making a positive choice towards something that we do want, rather than making a choice that is rooted in fear or is a reaction to something else. For instance, a woman may think she wants a home birth because she has been deeply affected by the story of a traumatic hospital birth that a friend told her some years ago. But, in reality, this may not be such a positive choice for her since it is based on the fear that she will experience similar trauma to her friend should she choose to birth in a hospital environment.

However, there is an opportunity for her to use this experience in another way. First, she could acknowledge the impact that the story has had on her and then use this as the impetus to find out more about birth in general. By ensuring that she is well-informed about birth she can then more freely choose the care and setting that will best support her in labour. On this journey, the woman may discover that relaxation is crucial in the first stage of labour since oxytocin, the hormone which causes the uterus to contract and the cervix to dilate, flows most easily when the sympathetic, the 'fight or flight', nervous system is not aroused. This may lead her to make a very personal choice about who and what she wants to include in her birthing environment – she knows herself better than anybody and only she can determine where and who with she will be most relaxed.

Decisions like this require self-reflection and ask us to make choices based on self-awareness. When we make autonomous, informed decisions that are in tune with our unique identity, there is no need to feel defensive – we know what our choices stem from and we know they are an authentic expression of who we are. These choices are neither 'right' nor 'wrong', they are just choices and they do not need to incorporate another person's judgements or preferences. There is nothing selfish about this way of choosing, since we hold equal respect for our choices and those of others.

When we make a commitment to a particular choice, it immediately awakens a sense of depth within us. It is energising and liberating and we can begin to support that choice with our behaviour and actions. Such focus opens new doors and a path unfolds before us which previously lay submerged. Suddenly, we get a feeling of what it is like to engage more deeply with ourselves and the world. For instance, a woman may be feeling confused about where to give birth – in a hospital delivery suite, a midwife-led unit within a hospital, a stand-alone birth centre, at home with an NHS midwife or an independent midwife, with or without access to a birthing pool, a combination of the above or even in the sea with dolphins swimming around her! But, not all of these options will be right for or available to her, so she needs to rule out what she doesn't want so that she can embrace what she does want. After doing some research and checking her body-feeling against the different options, the woman may choose a home birth. She may then start to feel very excited about this prospect and be filled with a new sense of purpose and enthusiasm for making it happen. Moreover, in sharing this journey with her partner, she may also bring about a new level of communication and cooperation in her relationship.

Once we have committed to a choice, whatever that is, it can cascade into a delicious pool of opportunity and support. When we engage with the world in the way that we want to, through active choice, it is cause for joy and celebration.

Exploring Choice In Pregnancy, Birth And Parenting

Throughout your pregnancy you will need to make numerous decisions about birth and parenting. Below is a list of some of things that you may want to think about – though not comprehensive, it covers most key areas. Cross out the ones you don't want to look at now. Then, make a commitment to explore three of the remaining items in detail. Once you have given your full attention to these three, you can slowly start to move onto the others.

Pregnancy

- Antenatal care
- Tests and scans
- Antenatal classes

- Diet and exercise
- Balance between work and rest
- Ways in which you and your partner will engage together with the pregnancy
- What work and social commitments you need to say No to in order to nurture your pregnancy
- Ways of meeting other pregnant women
- Sources of information about pregnancy, birth and parenting: books, films, websites, support groups etc
- Ways to make room in your life to connect with the growing baby

Birth

- Birth environment
- Birth attendants
- What you want to include in your birth plan/preferences (We'll look at this more closely in chapter five)

Parenting

- Baby's name(s), what surname will they take
- How you will engage with your family of origin and in-laws around the time of the arrival of the baby
- What visitors you do/don't want in the first few days and weeks, and what support you need from those visitors
- How you will build your postnatal support network
- Styles of parenting you would like to engage with
- How you feel about getting your baby into a routine versus being in tune with the natural rhythm of your baby's needs throughout the day
- How you will help your baby and family sleep restfully at night
- Childhood vaccinations

Truth

Working with No demands that we develop self-awareness. In doing so, we move into a higher state of consciousness, an awakening or enlightenment about who we are. As we do this, we are align ourselves with the universal spiritual laws of Truth. Most religions and spiritual practices believe that we should only treat others in a way that feels is right for ourselves, and treat ourselves in a way that feels right for others.

In this way, we are accountable only to ourselves, and therefore our actions, behaviour and words will reflect what is truthful for us in the present moment. This is what is called an expression of our authentic Self and, when done with consistency, strengthens our personal integrity. As our inner beliefs begin to shine through in our outer behaviour, we will feel a growing sense of power. This is helpful at any stage of life, but particularly during pregnancy, birth and parenting, a time when we can often feel very open and vulnerable – our hormones as well as our emotions play their part in this. The truth about No is that it helps make decisions around birth and parenting much easier, and helps us make choices that are more likely to support our way of being.

By allowing ourselves to relax into No, we can begin to understand how the external world is in so many ways a reflection what is going on in our inner world, and how easily our outer and inner worlds can sit together. This feeling of truth may instil us with a sense of wonder, a wondering about the essence of life and the bigger picture.

Even though pregnancy touches millions of women every second of the day, it is still seen as a miracle. But, it might not be until we conceive that we really begin to realise what this means. At the same time, as we become aware of the commonality of our experience and how it connects us with women all over the world and the rest of the humanity, we may also feel something shifting within us. This is not always easy to express. There are endless books and diagrams from which we can learn about the physiological aspects of pregnancy – how our body is changing and our baby is developing week by week – yet the more subtle processes of spiritual opening and awakening can be much more difficult to chart.

So, just as we choose to conceive or, if conception was unplanned, to maintain our pregnancy, we are exercising our free will and living from a place of Truth. In practising mindful choice, we can trust ourselves and be confident in our decisions. Truth and trust are our greatest ally in pregnancy and birth. With trust we can let go and surrender to the process. Truth asks us to come right back to ourselves. When we listen to and trust our inner wisdom or knowing, we avoid being distracted by others and their version of the 'truth'.

For many of us, trusting ourselves can feel strange or uncomfortable at first. So often Western society encourages us to put our trust exclusively in external sources of authority or expertise. However, by practising stillness and giving ourselves space to listen within, we gain a more lucid understanding of how to best serve our pregnancy and to birth our way. After all, no-one else has lived in this body with us for all these years. Only we know our own body intimately and only we know our baby with such intimacy. Trusting this, with a strong sense of where we end and our baby begins, we can make the best decisions for both of us in birth and parenting.

To be comfortable and confident with this process, it is imperative that we give ourselves time away from our busy schedule and agendas, at least for an hour or a part of a day each week, and really be with what's going on inside. To be with the more finite parts of ourselves – our boundaries, our identity, our choice, our truth – and work out how to nurture ourselves and baby. No is the express route to knowing ourselves, and if we know ourselves, we know how we want to birth. The most joyful birth is the one that is a true expression of who we are. As the saying goes, we birth how we live and we live how we birth.

Meditation On Truth

Deep within us lies a connection to truth. For some this comes as a loud and clear voice, for others it is a quiet and barely audible voice. For some, when all drops away, there is a Universal Truth in which we touch the unity of existence. No-one can define this for us and it is essentially something we need to experience rather than to philosophise. It may be helpful to consider two layers of truth. Firstly, personal truth. This is the place where we are free to express what feels right in choice and behaviour for us, in the present moment. It could be called instinct, or a deeper knowing. The second layer of truth is visible in those moments when we feel moved by something so much bigger than ourselves that we lose a sense of our individual self. During such moments we have a sense of joining with another, be it nature, another human being, a life force, an energy, Love or God.

To begin cultivating your connection to truth, practise this simple meditation on breath awareness to help still the busy mind and make spaces for a deeper sense of being to emerge. This is not complicated, all it requires is willingness.

Sit comfortably, perhaps on the floor with a wall behind you supporting your spine. Start by focusing your attention on your outbreath and allow it to help you to settle your body and mind. Feel yourself releasing tension in the body and feel yourself settling into the earth, deepening your contact with the ground, letting tightness and holding fall away from the hips, groin area, right through the big muscles of the buttocks. Now, invite in a sense of the ground coming up from beneath you, offering support. Notice where your body ends and the ground begins. As you continue to focus on the out-breath, have a sense of coming away from the front of your body, as if you are dropping back towards the back of your body, way back inside towards your spine. Let the front of your face and body become soft and empty and relaxed. Notice the moment's pause as the out-breath ends and you graciously wait to receive the inbreath. There is no need to grab, or to hurry the breath in. Just let it arrive. With your next outbreath, come back inside yourself once again. Continue with this for five to ten minutes, or for as long as feels comfortable. Notice and acknowledge thoughts as they arise and pay attention to those that are most loving and nurturing, as they are the ones closest to truth. Trust this inner voice.

Allow yourself to retreat to this inner place as often as possible during your pregnancy, wherever you find yourself – in the bath, in your bedroom, in nature – and notice when and where it feels most accessible. It will not only connect you with your baby, but it is also very useful practice for labour.

Case Study 1: *Sorry*

Emma and Darren

Approaching the birth of her third child, Emma was finding it difficult to release old resentments. Emma discovered that Sorry was a key word for her and that she felt pressure to get things right and be a good girl. Emma's midwife reminded her of her mother, and Emma felt that there was an expectation for her to be perfect when in fact Emma felt like a vulnerable young girl. Emma was unable to express her vulnerability, and so she was unsure whether or not she would be able to bring the whole of herself to her birthing.

Darren was also fearful about showing his vulnerability and felt that he was always expected to know what to do to make things right in any situation. This added to the drama of the relationship – Darren's response to Emma's fears was to spring into action and try to manage them which, by turn, infuriated Emma. Darren then experienced resentment because he felt that he was never good enough in Emma's eyes.

Firstly, we suggested that Darren took the pressure off himself to get it right, and instead simply listen to Emma with empathy and acknowledge her fears, rather than see them as a call to action. We also talked about how Emma could help Darren acknowledge his vulnerability.

Emma and Darren's daughter was born at home on their houseboat. Emma was able to approach her birth without the pressure to perform. Both Darren and Emma were able to relax and to work well together. The baby was born before the midwife arrived. Emma says: "I realised that I was in charge of my own birth. That it was mine, and that I didn't have to live up to anyone else's expectations. I no longer felt that I had to please other people, which gave me a great sense of power."

Darren felt less pressured and was able to respond to Emma's needs more easily, rather than reacting in a habitual way. "I had time to reflect and felt more liberated. I was more considered in my choices. It is harder to stop and pause, than it is to tread the path that is well-worn."

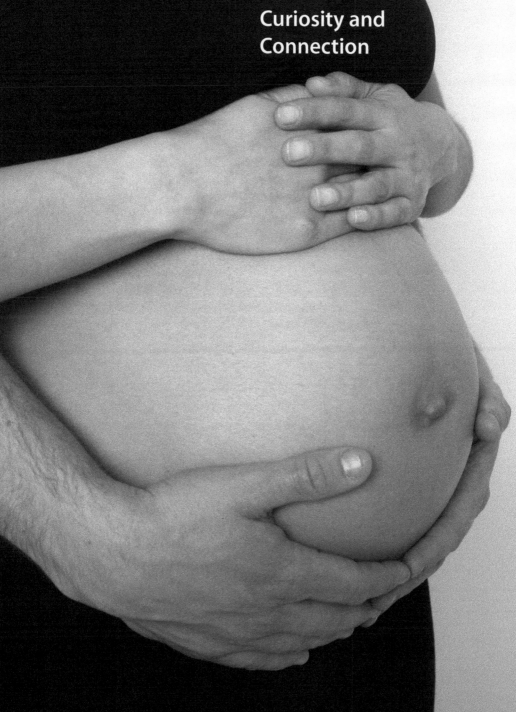

2 Hello

**Curiosity and
Connection**

If No helps us to nurture our identity, explore who we are and what is truthful for us in our lives, birth and parenting, then Hello ensures that we do not continue in isolation, but that we begin to engage and connect with those who can support us in this journey. So, the second secret of a joyful birth is 'Hello'. Hello awakens us to our natural curiosity in the world around us and the possibility of cultivating authentic communication between ourselves and others. It is about how we engage with our baby, with other pregnant women, our partner and with birth professionals; but it is also about how we connect with the true Self and about how open we are to the potential for birth and parenting to lead us towards a new understanding of ourselves.

Hello

Once we have established a healthy state of No, we can move towards others from a relaxed and grounded place. Since we feel confident about our identity, and respect the freedom with which others should be able to enjoy theirs, we can cast aside our steely defences. Having created such spaciousness around our lives, we then can embrace the state of Hello. Hello encourages us to cultivate a genuine curiosity in the world and to practice authentic communication. It is about interconnectedness. As we start to connect with and notice others, as we give and receive attention, then our relationships enter the realms of harmony and we experience a deep sense of being part of the whole.

New Realms

Clearly, in pregnancy, Hello expresses the essential need for us to acknowledge our babies as early as possible in their development – greeting and welcoming our babies into existence is the biggest Hello of all. But, Hello is also about the healthiness of being open to new ideas. Pregnancy takes us way beyond what we know in our lives. We can either approach this aspect of the journey with fear, contraction and control, or seize it as an opportunity to explore what else is out there. This will inevitably take us out of our comfort zone, but will ultimately lead us to new ideas that may be helpful and necessary.

Children bring about the potential to teach parents something profound about themselves, about their human-beingness, about their spirituality.

Experiencing Innocence

With Hello, we don't need to worry about making any decisions. We can simply enjoy noticing where we put our attention with the light-heartedness of a child. Often, we move through life in a habitual fashion, producing knee-jerk reactions to situations and repeating old patterns of behaviour. Pregnancy, however, is an occasion for us to delight in openness and exploration as we wander through different choices and discover new paths and directions.

For instance, we can choose to open our eyes and to see people as if for the first time. In this way we can glimpse who they really are. We can also choose to see ourselves and, of course, our babies, with such freshness. As we take nothing for granted and let go of our assumptions, we can take great pleasure in the world around us. By holding it lightly in this way, we will notice countless things that have evaded us before. Even if this is not our first pregnancy, we can celebrate it as a new journey, with another unique child. When we set out on any journey with such innocent awareness, we experience an abundance of opportunity, which enables us to move forward with the greatest sense of ease.

Opening To Ourselves

A pregnant woman's physiology supports this way of being too. During pregnancy, there is a magnificent cocktail of hormones flowing around our body, two of which are endorphins and relaxin. Endorphins are feel-good hormones, natural opiates and mood-enhancers, while relaxin has a softening effect on the body, helping to preparing it for the loosening and opening of the pelvis in birth. It also has a softening effect on the mind, so that we are less able to keep a lid on our emotions, similar to how a woman feels premenstrually. Thus we are physiologically designed to be more open in pregnancy than we would normally be in our non-pregnant state. By tuning into our body, by listening carefully to what it is telling us, we can learn to follow and trust our instinct, preparing ourselves at the deepest level for birth and parenting.

Breathing Life Into Relationships

A key aspect of Hello is communication. The couple relationship undergoes enormous changes with our first pregnancy, and experiences further greater changes with the arrival of additional siblings. Giving our relationship attention during pregnancy is crucial, as we may realise that the way we communicate with our partner may also need to change. By communicating in a non-aggressive manner, taking ownership of our needs and learning to stay open to the exchange, and listening in an active way, we can prepare and strengthen our relationship before the arrival of the baby. So, this baby and this birth can mark a new beginning for our relationship. Being open to this and being aware of how the quality of our communication can shape events, we can ensure that is a happy and enriching stage in our lives.

Keywords

Hello is about curiosity, openness, relationship and connectedness. From a clear state of No, we can begin to soften and to engage with the world in a playful manner, welcoming difference into our life without feeling defensive. In this way, we begin to change both what is internal and external and we become more connected to the whole. The four keywords of Hello, then, are: attention, openness, exchange; and communion. Let's explore how they could bring us to a more joyful experience of birth.

Attention

Our whole being seeks attention. It is like food for the soul. While it may be easy to criticise someone who is an 'attention seeker' for their extrovert behaviour – perhaps they are always creating a drama or trying hold other people's attention in an inappropriate way – it is not hard to see that it is precisely because they crave acceptance and interest from another human being that they act in this way. When we are heard by another with genuine acceptance and interest, it validates and helps us to make sense of our own experience. It also enables us to accept our humanness, so bringing with it feelings of relief and lightness.

As we embark on this new life with this new being, everyone involved needs to be mindful of what is happening, and mindful of each other. The new mother needs attention as she enters a period of monumental change, as does the father. It is often acknowledged that men want to be more involved, yet antenatal classes and culture still predominantly focus on the mother at the exclusion of the father. Dad should have plenty of attention and the opportunity to be actively involved in the pregnancy and birth, so that he has the confidence to do the same in his parenting. The baby in utero needs attention too, as its being comes into form and it prepares to makes its way into the world. It needs to feel held and loved in this process. Not any old kind of attention will do, though. It must be appropriate attention – so not needy, fear-based or narcissistic attention, but curious, non-judgmental, gentle and loving attention.

It is helpful to consider how we habitually give our attention to others. How do we give attention to ourselves, to our body and what it is telling us? How do we give attention to others? Do we really listen to people when they are talking to us? When we give partial attention we are only partially present or engaged. But when we give active attention, we are truly honouring ourselves and others. When we listen actively, we put our own agendas to one side and listen with 'big ears', noticing not only what someone is saying and the words they use, but also their body language and tone of voice. We might ask ourselves: 'What is this person telling me? What am I learning about them in this moment?' We notice any judgments as they emerge and let them go without a backwards glance.

If we never received appropriate attention in the early years, or if it was scarce, we may not expect or look for it as adults. Instead, we might replace it with improper substitutes that dull the senses and teach us little, feed us little. This may also mean we are not very good at giving attention to others, since we carry this hunger within ourselves. We may therefore come across as aggressive in our pursuit of attention or we may step back into a passive-aggressive state of self-pity and neediness.

Yet, how can we learn to not only to seek and enjoy good attention from others, but also to give it? The first thing is to begin by noticing how we feel when we are around someone who gives a certain presence of attention on a soul level. Notice how they listen and what they say. Then, we can start by giving someone else that same level of attention – we will look at this in more detail later in this chapter. As we become more practised at giving active attention, we can then begin to imagine what it would feel like to interact with everyone in this way, and to take that attention into other relationships in our lives.

As we bring our attention to those around us, it may also start to take a wider view and ask: Where do we put our attention with birth in this culture? As we did with No, we could look at what has so far informed us about birth – for, instance, antenatal classes, midwife appointments, friends and family, the media, our ethnic and cultural origin – and then begin to explore where we would like to put our attention in the future. There is no need to make a decision or commit to anything at the moment, we are simply interested in what's out there and in noticing what draws our attention.

Body Awareness

Make yourself comfortable – you could be relaxing in a warm bath or lying down on cushions. As you settle, begin by simply being aware of how your body rests on the bath or the ground. Can you soften the edges a little, letting go of the awareness of where you end and the ground begins, deepening into the support beneath you? Take your awareness to the ebb and flow of the breath, noticing it arrive and leave the body without you having to make anything happen. Just watch the natural, effortless cycle of the breath.

Now, what do you notice in your body? Are there any particular parts of your body that are calling out for attention? Perhaps there is a part of you that aches, or that feels tight or sore? Perhaps you have a sense of that part of the body being in need of something? If so, what would that be? What comes into your mind when you are connecting to this part of your body? Try visualising this part of you and listen to what it's saying, go in and really see what is there – don't worry about what comes forward, it could be anything. You might find yourself connecting with an emotion, a colour or a part of yourself that isn't getting enough room for expression. Move away from this part of the body and begin to roam freely around your body, giving high-quality attention and being open to what you find.

You can take this level of attention into your daily life. Be mindful of how your body feels within the pregnancy. Make a clear intention to listen to your body on a regular basis, really being open to what it is that your body wants to tell you – often our body can tell us what we need when our mind doesn't know. Are there particular symptoms of pregnancy that you notice? How does it feel in and around your pelvis? Your hips? Your womb? How does it feel around your lower spine, across the back of the pelvis? Can you allow softness to come into all these parts of your body as you gently bring your awareness to them?

When we are open to listening to our bodies, we will often find wisdom in unimagined places. Symptoms of pregnancy, nausea, heartburn, pelvic pain and so on, are all part of our pregnant journey. We could try and fix these symptoms rather than being open to and supporting them. But, by doing this we may lose out on an opportunity to know our bodies and ourselves better. So, next time you experience a symptom, bring your awareness to the feelings behind the symptom. What is the feeling behind the symptom? Is it irritation, fear or sadness? Some other quality of feeling or emotion? What other situations in your life can you recall when you have noticed this feeling? Can you bring a particular situation to mind? What was your habitual response in this situation? What is your habitual response to this symptom? What could you try differently that would serve you better and support you more? What can you learn about yourself from this?

Openness

From attention we move towards openness. If we are going to take something valuable from this journey and embrace everything that these new territories of pregnancy, birth and parenting have to offer, then we need to let go of our habitual ways of being. Most habits prevent us from trusting the world around us, which means that we are likely to remain in a closed, contracted way of being. Yet, by choosing to recognise our habitual responses, cast them aside for a moment, and instead be open and trusting of whatever comes along, then we may experience the world in a completely new way.

As we touched on before, many of us have not had a positive experience of attention. It may have been judgemental or controlling and we can therefore be wary of receiving or giving attention to this day. This prevents us from being open to new ideas. So, this aspect of Hello is about welcoming those new ideas and attitudes in, which is so helpful in pregnancy and birth, and sets us up for parenting. If we birth how we live, then pregnancy, birth and parenting are also about how we embrace the unknown and about how we trust and enjoy that process.

During our pregnancy, we need to be aware of our opinions – and hold them lightly, even if we have birthed before. Too many opinions can get in the way of being and relaxing into what is. Having an idea of what is important to us (our No) is one thing, but being fixed on the exact form of events is quite another. It will serve us well if we can get comfortable with saying 'I don't know' and bringing in a bit of 'we'll see as we go' into our lives and, as we explore our birth options, ask people around us, with genuine interest and acceptance, what they found useful in birth, what helped them.

By being curious, we may learn something from someone quite unexpected, which we then remember in labour and that really helps us to relax into birth and parenting. We never know who is going to teach us something really profound, and it is such a delight and a surprise when it comes from the person we least expected. Being in the world becomes so much more fun when we realise that every interaction is rich with potential and wisdom. Trust is essential to this way of being, just as it is essential to birth and parenting. If we are going to benefit fully from this life changing experience, then we need to let down our guard enough to trust.

In this way we can allow Hello to elevate our lives in ways we could hardly have dared to imagine. Pregnancy, birth and parenting are a journey of the highest order. When we go on holiday or to a different country we are often more open than when we are at home. Pregnancy may well feel like foreign territory at times, so we can approach it as such, as if we are visiting an unknown culture and country. In this way we can bring a sense of wonder, which enables us to appreciate difference without our usual sense of judgment. We need only take things moment by moment, not rushing ahead with plans and opinions.

Not only is it important that we nurture this sense of openness towards the world around us, but we also need to be curious about whether we feel able to bring attention to our baby in an open manner. That is, one that is without agenda and expectation. Can we easily choose to discard the internal commentary that chatters on: 'I want a son… a daughter… I want my son to be a lawyer or footballer or surgeon or… I want my daughter to be a doctor or model or actress or tennis star…' It is best to acknowledge these expectations with honesty – we all have them – and then let them go, so bringing ourselves to the far more fascinating job of being open. By doing so, we then open ourselves to the greatest capacity for joy in our birth and in our children. In this way our birth can be celebrated for its own unique experience, and our children can be celebrated for their own nobility and uniqueness.

Exchange

The third key word of Hello is Exchange, which is the realisation of our interconnectedness. While it is customary to exchange gifts, how often do we give and receive attention with complete openness? Yet when we do this, we expand our sense of Self by opening ourselves to the deep connection between every human being. Many cultures recognise this connection in their greetings to one another. The Mayans for instance, would say 'I am in You and You are in Me', while the Hindu salutation 'Namaste' translated simply means 'The God in me greets the God in you'.

In pregnancy, we rarely loosen ourselves to this kind of exchange with our baby. We often consider the baby to be 'taking' from the mother in a one-way stream. But, what exchange might there be in the other direction, from baby to mother? What might the baby being giving to its mother while in utero? Perhaps we could consider the possibility that the baby is giving its mother the gift of complete love, joy and acceptance, giving of itself and its experience without masking anything, and with utter openness, seeking to communicate with her in a very free way? Indeed, there are many ways in which the baby could be giving to its mother, yet in Western culture it is rare to acknowledge this. But, when we do acknowledge such exchanges, we make the baby real as a being, a being that needs to be seen just as it sees.

So, the biggest Hello in pregnancy is when the woman discovers she is pregnant. This is the time to appreciate the baby within, to say Hello and welcome its being into form. During the early stages of pregnancy, the baby's heart is beginning to develop and research shows that emotion may be enfolded within this organ even at such a young age. What emotions do we wish for our baby to enfold in its heart – shock, fear, rejection? Or pure love, joy and acceptance?

Some of a pregnant woman's initial reactions to the discovery of her pregnancy may get in the way of a clear, open Hello. But, there is always the opportunity to acknowledge these responses and then, once they have settled, lay them aside and say Hello to our baby in a way that is respectful and meaningful to the life within.

At this point, we may start to consider the question of when a soul enters a baby, if soul is indeed a possible part of our belief system. If the Soul does enter at the moment of conception, and some would say it is present even before conception, then what happens to that Soul when the mother – or father for that matter – does not acknowledge it when the pregnancy becomes known? And, even if our belief system struggles to accept a Soul in this way, is there a place for feeling and being responsive to the being growing within us? What kind of exchange would we like there to be, between mum, dad and baby, at this time?

Moving outwards, taking our attention away from the baby for a moment, there are other ways in which we might also explore Exchange. Primarily, we can return to the idea of active listening, which we mentioned before. Active listening is when we listen with big ears and a big heart, taking time to notice our own internal dialogue.

Everyone can lay claim to the fact that it is often all too easy to make assumptions about what the other person is saying, to think that we know what is being said, without taking proper care to really hear the other person's words, experiences and feelings, and to accept them for what they are. What's even more revealing is that we are most prone to this when we are in conversation with those people we are closest too, those we are related to, those we love. We think we know what they are saying before the words have come out of their mouths, or we switch off even before the moment they begin to communicate with us.

The way around this is, during conversation, to regularly come back to ourselves and to kindly question whether we are listening with those big ears and big heart – and to let go of any criticism of ourselves and our ability to listen. We can also use particular tools that will help us to check that we have heard the other person correctly, summarising what they have just said and beginning our sentences with the following phrases:

- 'It sounds like…'
- 'Do you mean…?'
- 'Are you saying…?'

(For more on active listening skills, see Listening To Ourselves, Listening To Others below.)

Opinions are not needed in active listening. Neither do we hi-jack the other person's experience by saying something along the lines of: 'I know exactly what you mean, that happened to me last Tuesday with so and so…' We can never assume that we truly understand what another person has experienced, and doing so gets in the way of authentic communication. Beyond the words, there is always a much deeper, more subtle tale being told and that requires careful, mindful attention in order to be heard. It is also very special to really hear and honour someone with active listening, and great levels of intimacy can ensue between the speaker and listener.

We can learn something about ourselves by listening and by being heard in this way, and we can learn something about our partner and close friends and family by listening and being heard in this way too. We may also learn something invaluable that touches our birthing and parenting. We are giving an amazing gift if we can nurture the intention to practise active listening with our baby, both in utero and once it is born. This isn't a difficult task, but it does require an open mind and a commitment to the possibility of true communication between two beings.

Connecting With Baby

Sit comfortably, either on the floor or on a chair, with support behind you for your back. Close your eyes and begin by focusing on the outbreath, allowing yourself to settle into the ground beneath you and having a sense of gently letting go with each outbreath. Sense where your body ends and the floor begins, then imagine one melting into the other.

Next, bring your awareness to the bottom of your spine and relax into it with each outbreath. Imagine the sacrum – the triangular bone at the base of your spine, which forms the back of the pelvis – becoming wider, softer, longer and more fluid. Allow that sense of relaxation to move gently up your spine, like warm water or a feeling of sunshine.

Now, start to take your awareness away from the front of your body, way back inside yourself. In this way, the front of your face, your heart space, your torso, somehow become emptier, quieter and more relaxed. As you drop back inside yourself, towards your spine, perhaps you can find the true meaning of the word 'laid-back' by resting back inside yourself.

From this rested, laid-back place, begin to take your attention towards your baby, or babies. Your baby is basking in the radiance of your being. Can you bring the same sense of openness and awareness that you have just given your body, to your baby? Can you acknowledge that there is a human being within you that has chosen you as its first step towards being in this world? Your baby hand-picked you as its mother.

Your baby listens to every part of your being – the sound of your heart beat, the song of your breath, the gurgles of your digestive system, the rhythm of your daily routines. What can you sense about your baby? What can you notice about them as an intelligent, feeling, knowing being?

Hang out here for a while with your baby, just being gently curious about this little person. How are they doing? What might you learn about their world? Let go of any assumptions or judgments about yourself or your baby. There is no right or wrong here. This is simply the meeting of two people, at the beginning of a long journey together, starting to gradually get to know each other.

When you are ready, let your baby know you are going to take your attention away from them. Reassure them that you will return with full attention before too long. Let your baby know that it is seen and loved in all its glory, and you can apologise if this feels difficult.

Bring your awareness back to your breath for a few cycles of the breath. Then allow yourself to gently return your awareness to the outside world, opening your eyes and moving gently when you are ready, and in your own time.

Communion

At its most subtle level, when we embody Hello, we say Hello to the Divine, whatever that means to us as an individual – and the Divine says Hello back through the eyes of another. Every interaction has the potential to reveal something to us about ourselves and the nature of all things. This invitation is always available to us and, through this understanding, we can gain a sense of how that which we experience and notice in the world reflects the attitudes and perceptions of our interior world.

Since we have already strengthened our chosen identity by working with No, we can be more mindful of where we put our attention in Hello. Externally, we are opening our eyes to see how the world around us chooses to puts its attention on pregnancy, birth, babies and parenting. From here, we can then invite in different and new experiences, welcoming them in as a possibility for ourselves, and in doing so we will begin to notice a growth in our being, which is both palpable to ourselves and others.

Allowing ourselves to rest lightly in Hello, we bring the grace of communion into our lives. That grace could be with a partner, our baby, with friends, family, with other mothers and fathers, or with nature. We are not fixing on any single experience, but celebrating an attitude that opens us to the beauty and joy of the world – and of pregnancy, birth and parenting – in all its glory.

Birth is part of the natural cycle of life and death, and we can learn much from nature about birth. Watching nature films that explore birth can therefore be incredibly helpful as we prepare for our own birth. Nature has the ability to reveal to us the rawness and simplicity of birth free from the tumultuous hype that we humans tend to create around the process. No mammal would need books or antenatal classes to help them birth freely.

In nature, we can witness the basic interaction of hormones and the beauty of mammalian physiology at work, unhampered by the uber-developed neo-cortex of the human brain. While viewing, we could ask: What can I learn about myself as I observe my reactions to these programmes? Where can I most easily put my attention? What bits are most difficult for me to focus on? Is it somehow easy for me to see the wonder of birth in nature, yet less easy for me to see how that might relate to my own birth?

Nature reflects not only the experience of birth in humans, but the experience of pregnancy too. During pregnancy, the woman undergoes a natural, metaphorical process of maturation. She is like a sun kissed gourd who, unseen, mysteriously ripens from the inside out. Her hormones assist her in this process, relaxin softening both her ligaments and pelvic area, as well as her emotions. This has the effect of enabling the woman to let down her defences – and, when she engages her partner in the process, for him to do so to – and so both can become available to the baby in a more whole, connected way. From this place, she and her partner can welcome the baby without agenda, as a seed full of potential and bursting with its own interminable life force. The wonder and curiosity with which we regard nature can clearly be an ally in our own lives, helping us to arrive at our parenting in a ripe and fruitful place.

Finally, in communion, we can recognise that much of the longing for relationship and contact, or hunger for attention, is derived from a deep yearning for contact with the Divine. Communion asks us to sit within this realm, a realm in which we acknowledge the sacred both within us and outside of us, within another. There is a sublime sweetness in this kind of relationship, a relationship in which all needs are sated, and all expectations have been replaced by acceptance.

So, let us take this communion, this heartfelt sense of interconnectedness, into our relationship with our baby. Let us see the divinity within the baby inside us, accept the baby as a human being on a Soul level from the earliest possible moment and, moreover, entertain the idea that our babies see the whole of us, in the fullness of our being, and without judgment. Can we honestly meet our babies in this place? If so, we have truly opened ourselves to the second secret of a joyful birth.

Listening To Ourselves, Listening To Others

In previous exercises, we explored ways of opening to communication with your body, and then with your baby. So, now let's look at how you can bring that openness into relationship, with the people you encounter as you make your way through pregnancy, birth and parenting. A fundamental way of doing this is through active listening.

Active listening is a skill that you can choose to use when and wherever an obvious need arises; not necessarily when you're engaged in general chit-chat or small talk. Perhaps it is most useful when you begin to talk about something either you or your partner feels is important. Indeed, there may be many 'important conversations' when you are pregnant. Be attentive to this. It is not always easy to define what is important or not to someone else – and they may not always see what's important for you. It may therefore be helpful to say when you are bringing something to a conversation that you feel needs proper attention. Be aware of difference; allow yourself and your partner to express your differences, differences in opinion, in preference and in ranking importance.

So, the first thing you do when you practise active listening is to make a mental note that you are consciously moving into that space. In this way, you become 'all ears' and so you may occasionally need to check that you have not misheard (easy to do) or made an assumption (also easy to do). This is a valuable thing to do during your antenatal appointments, as well as with significant others.

First of all check that you have understood what the other person has said. Ask: 'Do you mean…?' or 'Is what you're saying…'. The next step, one which may feel much harder, is to question what judgments and clutter we are bringing to the conversation – you'll recognise it by that internal chatter that gets in the way of open listening. Pause yourself when you start saying things like: 'Well, I don't agree with that…', 'You're wrong, I can remember what happened when…', 'You never understand…', or 'I wouldn't do it like that!' The point is to listen to what the other person is saying, not to what your opinion is on that.

It's not easy to master, but there is a special quality to active listening. Holding yourself back from expressing opinions, giving advice and ticking the other person off, can be a huge challenge. So, to counteract such irresistible urges to bring in your own ego, it can be helpful to instead concentrate on posing open-ended questions to the speaker. For instance, 'So what do you want to do with that?' 'Where does that leave you?' or 'Where will you go from here?'

Obviously, if you are listening to your antenatal care attendants or midwife, these questions may not be relevant. Nevertheless, it is always useful to clarify what has been said so that you don't leave having misheard and then misinterpreted some vital piece of information. Once you are clear about what has been said, then you can be clear in your response – rather than reacting to something that wasn't clearly communicated in the first place.

When you do feel the need to respond, use an 'I' statement, rather than a 'You' statement that directs fault at the other person. For example, sentences that begin 'You always…' or 'You never…' are not helpful. Instead, go for something like: 'I notice I struggle with that… I wonder why?' or 'I notice I love it when you do, or say…' It is much more constructive to opt for open communication around what you notice rather than blameful allegations about what you perceive as the ways in which the other person has let you down.

The key is to take absolute responsibility for the way you communicate so that you can glide through clear waters, rather than flounder in the murky depths of muddy communication.

Finally, before you put down this chapter and go into the

outside world again, take some time to ask yourself a few questions, and answer them honestly.

- How open are you when your partner is trying to tell you something? What kind of internal chatter do you hear?
- How open are you when you chat to other pregnant women who are making different birth choices to you?
- When do you feel most able to converse in a light-hearted manner with others?
- What does your culture focus on in birth and parenting?
- Where is your attention most easily drawn in pregnancy?
- Where do your friends and pregnant peers put their attention in relation to birth?
- How useful do you find it listening to other women about their pregnancy and birth experiences?
- From where are you acquiring your knowledge of birth and pregnancy? Is it from pregnancy classes, midwives, TV, or friends or family?
- How could you open yourself to information about birth that is different to that which you have previously focused on?
- What do you know about other cultures and their birthing practices?
- Where could you find out about other birthing practices – for instance, about home birth, midwife-centre birth, hospital birth, lotus birth, different kinds of birth support…?
- Could you ask your midwife and other local pregnant women for information about groups and classes happening in your area that you may not have heard about?
- How open are you to accepting your baby may be having a different experience from you right now?

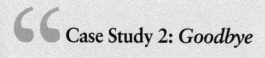

Case Study 2: *Goodbye*

Sophie

Pregnancy is a time of transition and Sophie was struggling to step out of old roles. She felt that she was a carer to her mum and sisters, and that she had to attend to their emotional needs and take care of everything. With her first pregnancy Sophie was being drained by this role and realised that it was not helping her transition into motherhood. Sophie felt that she needed to be looked after, or at least for there to be a recognition that she had needs too.

Sophie began to explore ways of communicating with her family. She decided to begin by telling her mother that she intended to have a home birth. Sophie had not told her mum before because she didn't want her to worry and become overly anxious. Sophie also decided that she needed to speak to her sister and explain that she could no longer provide the level of support she had previously been giving her as she now needed to direct some of that energy towards looking after herself. Sophie's mum responded well, but her sister was not so receptive. However, Sophie felt that this was OK and that it was not appropriate to keep rescuing her sister. Communicating in this way gave Sophie a sense of space and relaxation and she was more able to be with her baby and partner.

Sophie went two weeks over her due date, during which she became fed up and uncomfortable. She agreed to induction on day 16. The day before her induction was booked, Sophie had a big cry and let go of her desire to have a home birth – for her birth to be a certain way. She had to say Goodbye to what she had hoped for and she had to accept that she did not want to wait any longer. This letting go was powerful enough for her to clear the way for her birth and she went into labour spontaneously that night.

During the morning Sophie had a bleed and her midwives said that they would prefer it if she laboured in hospital. Again, Sophie had to let go in herself of the possibility of a home birth and was able to be clear about what she needed to do. Sophie's baby was born in hospital and she felt great joy around her birth. She said that birth had allowed her to go through a process of peeling away the layers of her past and let go. Goodbye had given a structure within which to work with this process. Sophie said that during each contraction she said Goodbye to the pain with each out breath, and that this enabled her to trust more deeply in her journey towards motherhood.

"

3 Thank You

Remembering Love

A wise man once said that the journey of the pregnant woman is to grow her heart as big as her uterus. In this way pregnancy is about attending to both our emotional and spiritual needs, as well as our physical needs – like a ripening gourd, much of our maturing and mellowing occurs within and cannot be witnessed from the outside. The third secret of a joyful birth, saying Thank you, is about recognising that nourishing the heart of a pregnant woman and her baby is as important as nourishing her body. Indeed, in many other cultures a woman's uterus is often referred to as her second heart, with the understanding that what we hold in our heart we hold in our womb, and what we hold in our womb we hold in our heart. For instance, within the Japanese hands-on healing tradition of Shiatsu, the heart-womb meridian is seen as vital for healthy conception, pregnancy and birth, and so a strong connection between the two is given particular attention when treating a woman at this stage in her life.

Thank You

So how can Thank you bring us more joy in our birthing? In the previous chapter, Hello, we began to cultivate an awareness of where and how we place our attention in the world, in relationship and with our baby, thereby strengthening feelings of interconnectedness and gaining confidence in our ability to communicate openly and authentically. With Thank you we can start to refine this way of being further, by bringing ourselves back to our hearts, the resting place of the Self, and so moving from the foundation of honest exchange towards a deepening of our connections through gestures of heartfelt appreciation for ourselves and others. By experiencing the pleasure that this can bring us in our pregnancy, we can learn to trust more and thereby enter our births with an open heart. As we will discover, it is when we birth with our hearts, not our heads, that we really empower ourselves to birth in a way that supports the natural release of the most important birth hormones – oxytocin, the love hormone, and endorphins, the feel-good hormones – and is thus potentially less arduous and more joyful.

As always, however, we mustn't forget to be gentle with

ourselves in this process. For many of us, baby steps may be best as, at first, trusting and acting from our hearts may feel uncomfortable. Generally, Western culture does not encourage us to live in a heart-centred way, a way of life that was probably more accessible to us as children. Adult life is busy and pressured, and fear rather than trust often predominates. What's more, in the past, we may have defended our heart for what appeared to be good reason, and so we might need to recognise that it will take time to drop our defences as we start to support and nurture the more vulnerable parts of ourselves. What's so wonderful in pregnancy though is that, if we are open receiving their help, our baby is there with us, helping us do whatever we need to make that opening happen.

Loving Relationships

Inevitably, Thank you has everything to do with relationship, since it is a practice that reveals many ways in which we can learn about the nature of love and family. In pregnancy, Thank you touches upon our relationship with our self, our changing body, our baby as it grows within us, and our relationship with this baby's father. Thank you may then present a challenge to us, asking us to consider how we are in relationship. Perhaps we enter into relationship with the burden of blame and criticism, appropriating the language of a culture that shies away from personal responsibility? Or perhaps we bring so many expectations to every relationship, including our relationship with our self that it is hard for us to appreciate someone simply for who they are and what they bring? However we do relationship, though, it is heart-warming to know that the remedy for our faults is not to do ourselves in with self-criticism, but to love ourselves more. The heart gets stronger with gentle care, responding quickly to loving attention – and when we learn to care about the state of our own heart; we will spontaneously start to care more about the state of others'.

We can love ourselves on a practical level through nourishing ourselves with wholesome food, much-needed rest, soulful music and a calming environment. We can also do this on an emotional and spiritual level through caring for our relationships and developing trust. We may well notice that we feel better about who we are when we are around certain people, because of the way they treat us, speak to us, care for us. Likewise, there's no doubt that there are certain people who feel better about who they are when they are around us. As a gesture of commitment to understanding our own heart journey better, we can begin to notice these exchanges and the aspects of our relationships that are blessed with such love. In relationship to ourselves, meanwhile, we can notice when we are engaged with activities or in situations that bring about a sense of true relaxation – an active relaxation, not a collapsing into a heap relaxation. With true relaxation comes restedness, well-being and a sense of being at ease in your own skin.

Child's Play

The state of Thank you is one that is often embodied more easily by children rather than adults, through displays of innocence and natural kindness. Rather than approaching relationships and the day heavy with expectation, guilt and defensiveness, children are often able to approach the unknown with a sense of excitement and pleasure. In reconnecting with that effortlessness with which a young child expresses their love, Thank you may help us to clarify what we value, what feels really good deep inside, and may lead us to a level of appreciation previously unknown to us.

There is always room for more appreciation in pregnancy and birthing, and we should take every opportunity to step away from cloying negative language about how tiring and draining pregnancy is, how painful and traumatic labour can be, how exhausting and draining it is to care for a young baby. Of course, there is a place for naming our struggles and fears and having them validated, but there is also a place to acknowledge what is good and blessed in our life. Fostering gratitude in our daily lives can bring so much more joy to our pregnancy – and it would be a shame to take pregnancy for granted, since it is not a journey we go on very many times in our life, and it is always a privilege.

Keywords

There are many ways in which we can say Thank you – in conversation, with a kiss, a notecard, a gift. But, when we pay more attention to what is expressed when we say Thank you, we find that it holds many different aspects of ourselves. In a sincere Thank you we find: appreciation, an affirmation of another person's uniqueness; valuing, raising something or someone above other things or people in our lives; giving, both a heartfelt response and a letting go; and, heart essence, an awareness of how the giving and receiving of unconditional love can be deeply touching. By taking some time to consider Thank you in its fullness, we can get closer to our hearts and, by knowing our hearts more fully, we can birth more wholly and with greater joy.

Appreciation

When we really appreciate something or someone, we provide affirmation of those special qualities that make them unique. We choose to acknowledge something that we see in them which is particular to them. Within each of us is a yearning to be appreciated in this way and it touches that innocent childlike place in which we are seen in our goodness. It warms the heart. It touches us. A simple gesture of appreciation can bring about tears. It means someone has noticed us or what we do. When someone receives appreciation, they may feel more valued not only by others, but by themselves. It gives them permission to love themselves a little more. From the simple act of saying Thank you we can have a very profound effect on others.

For a baby in utero, the experience of being appreciated may have an enormous long-term effect on the shaping of their soul. To be surrounded in love and appreciation from such an early age, means that right from the beginning of its life the baby can relax into a place that feels good, warm and full of heart. It reflects the baby's own goodness back to them, and creates a sense of well-being and harmony that enhances their growth and development.

During experiments in which mothers played music to their baby throughout their time in the womb, new born babies responded most strongly to the music that their mothers had enjoyed the most.

Significantly, when a mother listened to music she loved it was not only pleasurable for her, but also for her baby. When a pregnant woman truly appreciates something, she releases the feel-good hormones endorphins that are a gift to baby too. It's important, then, that we spend at least some of our pregnancy engaged in activities and with people that we enjoy. Things that will feed and nourish us on a heart and soul level. Both mother and baby benefit from such commitments. So, taking time to notice and feel into what we appreciate at this time in our life is a marvellous use of time. It shows we appreciate our Self, our pregnancy, our baby.

It is those feelings of appreciating or being appreciated that make the difference. It is sensing the heartfelt quality, a quality that is more than just words. When we experience true appreciation, then it is almost as if it awakens a memory within us that helps us to remember who we are – and us humans are often in the habit of forgetting who we really are. True appreciation feels good, like taking a warm bath. Indeed, it is exactly these kinds of simple gestures that nourish us within our daily lives.

When we act on a feeling of appreciation, either verbally or through gesture, it becomes something more than simply existing as an internal feeling. It pushes that feeling out, gives it form, and helps us to be more authentic. When we express appreciation verbally yet are pandering to expectation and don't really mean it, our tone of voice and body language give us away. Gestures, therefore, need to be sincere, rooted in the body, if they are to convey a deeper meaning.

Some people find appreciating themselves and others easy. Yet, not being appreciative can be a habit. Some people may grow up in a family in which showing appreciation is not part of their everyday lives and so may not learn its value. If this has been the case, then we should challenge ourselves to be appreciative, even if it feels forced or tentative to begin with. Always looking for what is wrong with a person or situation can be a default response. For instance, it might be easier for us to complain about our pregnancy symptoms than to embrace the excitement and to acknowledge all the other kinds of feelings that may be bubbling beneath the surface, eager to be expressed.

We need to recognise what we are struggling with, sure, but we also need to avoid getting stuck in that place. We need to ask: What else is there? Where is there place for more appreciation in my life? In this way, we are less likely to take anything or anyone for granted and we can start to be more aware of our feelings of gratitude.

Bringing Heart And Appreciation Into Your Life

If you can make a it a daily practice to offer gestures of appreciation then everyone, including yourself and your baby, will benefit. Firstly, take nothing for granted, ask your partner what gestures from you would help make them feel appreciated – it can be easy to make a wrong assumption here. Then share with them the kinds of gestures which work for you. These could be anything from a cup of tea in bed in the morning, to running a bath with oil and surrounded by candles to bringing home good food or receiving a massage at the end of the working day. Then, commit to making three gestures, unprompted, each week. Now, turn your attention to your baby. Commit to giving baby a daily gesture of appreciation – sending them your love, saying 'hi', taking a moment to be curious about their development and validating their experience, even if you are not sure what that is, or playing music you love to your baby every day.

Pregnancy, birth and parenting are all about love. So, through these gestures of appreciation create an environment in your home that nurtures important relationships. This takes courage, and courage works well in alignment with trust. You must learn how to look after yourself in this way, as it is not something you'll learn through modern antenatal care – your midwife or obstetrician is highly unlikely to say 'get the love flowing and look after your heart', though many other people who work with birthing women may. Seek people who help you bring feelings of warmth and relaxation into your life. It will do much in helping you to prepare for birth, for being parents, and it will do so much more than any book in the world will ever do for you. Take heart!

Valuing

If we acknowledge what we value with truth and integrity, then our actions will be in alignment with our thoughts, and we will have a stronger sense of identity. We all see the world in different ways, and we place different value on different people and different situations. When we allow ourselves to value something, then we raise it up in our estimation by giving it specific attention and holding it with greater regard than those things which we have not chosen to value in that moment. By turn, we all offer our thanks differently, and by doing so we each express something of who we are. Thus, in pregnancy and parenting, what we choose to value along the way will tell us a great deal about who we are as individuals, as parents, and what is and isn't important to us. This asks us to make considered and heartfelt choices.

For instance, we might hear ourselves say that we value natural birth yet put little or no time into making use of networks and classes which support this idea, choosing instead to channel our energy into decorating the nursery and buying baby clothes and toys. But, it's not about making judgements about what or where we choose to put our time and money. Instead, we need to check that our actions are actually in alignment with our thoughts. This helps us to be clear about what we really value – and what our partner really values too.

We often need to check to see whether we value everything we do have around us, rather than valuing what we don't have – are we a grass is always greener kind of person, or can we value where we're at? Within the couple relationship, it is more helpful to focus on what our partner does bring to the relationship, rather than focusing on areas in which we perceive lack or feel let down. Likewise during the transitional stage of pregnancy, it is helpful to focus on it as a fruitful time – an opportunity to grow, learn something new about ourselves, expand our ability to give and receive love, bring some resolve and integration to past hurts, and more – rather than clinging to our previous life or feeling restricted by our pregnant body.

Couples can learn a lot about each other through conversations about what each partner values in this pregnancy, this birthing, this parenting. There will be differences, but accepting that we value different things and finding a way to nurture each other in this journey is part of the challenge – and, if Dad could grow his heart as big as his partner's uterus, then that would be incredibly helpful and baby would certainly benefit too! Working from the heart, allows for a quality of open-mindedness that serves a new soul best. It is an enormous gift to receive a child, and valuing and trusting this soul is the least we can do. Not everyone who would like to have a child is able, and this should remind us that we cannot take pregnancy and parenting for granted.

When we say Thank you, both the giver and the receiver are elevated to a place of value. Both people feel-good and are touched by the experience. In noticing something about someone, and then valuing that quality of action enough to say Thank you, you offer the possibility for that person to grow bigger within themselves, perhaps allowing a part of them more room for expression than had previously been given. When you notice that special something in someone, it is like taking a tiny seedling and transplanting it into more fertile soil, moist with potential. So, imagine what it must be like for a tiny baby within its mother to experience that quality of attention, to be given such a nurturing environment in which to grow. The simple act of saying Thank you, therefore, is like a flowering. It brings beauty and radiance to life.

Giving

Giving is a natural response from the heart. In giving, we relax, we let go of holding. Miserly people are often also described as 'tight'. So, practising the opposite, giving freely from the heart, may literally loosen us up. When a pregnant woman is able to find an authentic place within herself from where she can give freely to her baby – give love, attention, appreciation – then, without knowing, she will have also found a place from which she can help prepare her body for labour. In birth, the body has soften so that our baby can be born and we must let go emotionally and physically in a way that we have perhaps never done before.

Our partners can help us soften too. A partner who is able to regularly give to their partner with heartfelt ease, helps the pregnant woman to let go since we also need to soften in order receive, not just to give. Moreover, giving and receiving increases those feel-good hormones, endorphins, which we already know benefit both mum and baby. Meanwhile, another hormone is at work, relaxin, the main purpose of which is to support softening during pregnancy. Relaxin is released throughout pregnancy and gradually relaxes all the smooth muscle and ligaments in the body so that our pelvis and pelvic floor are eventually soft and open enough to birth our baby.

Indeed, the physiology of labour is powered by hormones, not only relaxin and endorphins but also, crucially, oxytocin, the love hormone. Oxytocin, which stimulates the uterus to contract, is the same hormone that floods a woman's body (and a man's, for that matter) when she makes love. Oxytocin flows at conception, birth and in breastfeeding and is a mother's best friend.

In the first stage of labour, when the contractions open the cervix, pulling it up around the baby's head so that the way is clear for it to pass into the birth canal and be born, the flow of oxytocin is helped by the arousal of the para-sympathetic nervous system, just as during lovemaking. As well as oxytocin, endorphins are easily released when we are feeling safe, loved, trusting and able to express ourselves, free of inhibition. This is the realm of the older, primitive brain and it comes into its own when we can quieten the newer, thinking (or neo-cortex) brain. As in matters of the heart, in romance and lovemaking, if we activate the thinking brain during labour and birth it will dampen the mood and prevent us from going with the flow.

When a woman orgasms, however, she excites the sympathetic nervous system and adrenalin, the fight or flight hormone which would not previously have been conducive to proceedings, comes into its own. There is a flush, a climax, a release. The same occurs in birth. As a woman moves into transition, the period between the first stage of contractions to the pushing stage when baby is born, she may often express fear, uncertainty and appear to reach the limits of her ability to cope. Pioneering French obstetrician, Michel Odent, describes this physiological fear as necessary for the woman to birth her baby. The adrenalin begins to flow and it provides the woman with the

Discovery

Exactly at the time when most of us discover we are pregnant, around six weeks, the baby is busy growing a huge heart. In fact, the baby is pretty much all heart. So it helps to be mindful of how we relate to this being at this time.

If the news of your pregnancy was a shock and there was ambivalence and ambiguity around being pregnant, then start by acknowledging, without guilt, that your baby may have experienced this in the form of stress hormones and peptides (hormones which carry emotions). Then, encourage your baby to let go of this and ask them to accept your apology for not being as ready to receive the news as you would have liked. Then, welcome them with love and appreciation and let them know how much you value this pregnancy and their coming into the world. Thankfully, there is always the choice for us to go back and take responsibility for the times at which our experience may have impacted another.

impetus to release her baby, with the help of powerful, expulsive contractions.

In the first stage of labour we must go with the flow, in transition we face our darkest fears, and then in the second stage we come to the biggest letting go of our lives in order to give birth to new life. In this way, a woman has to find a depth of trust within her that she may never have felt before. This is love and complete surrender in action.

While this level of surrender is a great gift to baby in itself, we can give to the baby on a still deeper level by acknowledging the baby during birth. This means accepting that the baby is also with the intensity of labour, connecting with them and validating their experience at this time. This is not just a gift that a mother can give to her baby by keeping the baby in her mind while birthing, but one that her partner and birth attendants can give too, by communicating with and encouraging the baby through labour and birth.

So, giving gives form to feeling. It provides clarity where there may have been confusion and ambiguity. When we give to someone, that person has a better understanding of our feelings. We can give in many ways that will help prepare us to give fully in birth, and we can practise this in pregnancy by giving a listening ear to a friend, a back rub to our partner, a delicious meal cooked with love. Simple gestures such as these are worth so much. When your feelings are expressed through action, the receiver feels remembered, valued, cared for and loved. Giving in this way is unconditional, there is no expectation of reward or exchange. The pleasure comes from knowing that the other person will feel-good and that you have been able to extend them your love.

Giving is like a magical power through which we can make a difference. We can help transform the feelings of the receiver. This is the responsibility that comes with giving. We must consider how the gift clearly demonstrates our feelings, however small that gift may be. We must also put ourselves in the shoes of the receiver to imagine what is the right gift for them so that it fits with that person and enhances their sense of Self.

It might also be about gifting ourselves, as a way of honouring our pregnancy and transition into parenthood. For instance, we might feel that, even though it may take time away from the family, we need to gift ourselves with good teachers and studies that support our own learning and passions in life, so that we can be the best parents we can be. Gifting ourselves in this way, means that we can feel excited in our journey as parents. If something feels good and healthy in nourishing us a new parent, we should do it. We all need to look after own hearts, so that we can better care for those of our children.

Heart Essence

In growing our heart as big as our uterus, we can see how important it is to relate to our pregnancy in a heartfelt way. Certainly, from the earliest awareness of pregnancy, it is essential that we relate to our baby with heart. From the moment we discover we are pregnant, or as soon as we become aware of the need to acknowledge our baby in this way, we need to realise that our baby grows best in a womb with

70

a mother who looks after her sense of heart. Simply reminding ourselves that there is a sentient and vulnerable being within us who deserves to be treated with love and respect, whatever is going on, is a huge beginning.

Children are among the best teachers of unconditional love, which is what we mean when we talk about heart essence. Unconditional love is the kind of love that is not dependent on anything. This is the highest form of love, but it's not always easy to give. So, how can we free ourselves to learn to give in this way?

Knowing ourselves and accepting ourselves in all our humanness is a good start. The more we accept and know ourselves, including the murky bits and the less appealing aspects, the more we have capacity to accept others in their humanness. As always, the journey starts with our self. What aspects of love and relationship do we find hard to engage with? Where do we struggle with self-acceptance? Through gently self-enquiry we can start to understand our responses to situations and the ways in which we express love, thereby bringing less of an agenda to our birthing and parenting. Ultimately, it makes more space for us to follow our heart and go with the flow.

Letting go of self-judgment can feel like a monumental task for many of us, yet as long as we continue to judge ourselves, we will also judge others, including our children. Self-acceptance teaches us a lot about unconditional love, since by loving ourselves – as opposed to constantly pushing for more change, for betterment – we allow ourselves to shine more brightly and for our love to pour forth. This is love indeed. Some would go so far as say that love is at the root of our human experience, that any human action is either an extension of love or a cry for love, that those are the only two truthful choices in our lives.

There is a simplicity in open-hearted love. It doesn't need to define itself or the conditions attached to it; there are none, it just 'is'. Unconditional love, the expression of our heart essence, feels delightful to both the giver and the receiver. It has a fierce strength and freedom to it which knows no bounds; a courage and willingness that nourishes even the darkest corner, bringing warmth to the coldest chill, like balm to the soul.

We can ask ourselves: What makes it easiest in my pregnancy for me to connect with my heart? When are I most likely to feel warm and trusting and in alignment with my truth? Where do I feel most clarity in my life? What gets in the way of that? Fear and unresolved issues from the past are a common block to love (more on this in chapter six).

For now, let's see if we can sense an unconditional love within us easing out the creases, bringing relaxation and sensitivity. See our baby from this place, a hugely radiant yet vulnerable being who has come here to experience human life and hand-picked us as the perfect teachers. By opening our hearts to see this being, we acknowledge the presence of a beautiful and intricate piece of the universe. There is a miracle taking place right here right now, in the exchange of two human beings, one body inhabiting the other. How often do we have the privilege of being part of such a joyful event?

Nurturing The Heart-Womb Connection

Strengthening the connection between the heart and the womb, known as the Heart-Womb meridian or energy channel in Eastern medicine, can help us to get the most from our pregnancy and birth. The woman's uterus is often regarded as her second heart in many cultures and the two are inextricably linked – what you hold in your heart, you hold in your womb, and vice versa. A strong flow, or connection, between the two, therefore, strengthens a woman's internal resources for pregnancy and labour. It also helps to keep the heart open. You can nurture the heart-womb meridian in a number of ways:

- Sit comfortably, with support if needed, close your eyes, place one hand on your heart and one hand on your belly, and visualise the connection between your heart and your womb. From here, you could bring your awareness to your breath and then imagine as if you were breathing first from the heart, and then from the womb, and then both simultaneously.

- Again, sitting comfortably, with one hand on your heart and one hand on your womb, close your eyes and chant 'MA', which is said to be the sound which nourishes the heart-womb meridian.

- Drink lemon-balm tea.

- Enjoy a massage using melissa essential oil, which is derived from lemon-balm.

Meditation On Unconditional Love

Trust is the foundation of loving relationships and so we need to do everything we can to nurture feelings of trust in our lives. Begin by trusting in the rightness of your pregnancy. This baby chose you, no-one else. It has made a wise choice. Allow yourself to get a sense of how that feels.

Sit or lie in a position that is comfortable and supported. Settle into your body and gently become aware of the ebb and flow of the breath. Have a sense of coming back inside yourself, away from the front of your body towards your centre. Feel into your womb and begin to acknowledge the presence of your baby. Imagine the baby basking in your being. Imagine them as they see you in all your glory and enjoy the warmth of that feeling. Imagine them accepting you unconditionally as their mother, the mother they chose above every other.

Now, see if you can begin to see your baby in that way, as a being who shines such a bright light within you that you can receive the love and warmth that your baby emanates and extends towards you. Let baby's love envelop you in anyway it wants to, and then envelop your baby in your love, allowing it to flow freely from your heart and surround the entirety of their being. Trust in love.

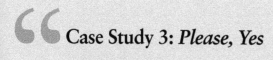

Case Study 3: *Please, Yes*

Lisa and Tom

Lisa and Tom had found the birth of their first child in Holland very traumatic. They had planned a home birth but were transferred to hospital, where Lisa felt that she was treated with neither care nor respect.

Working through the Seven Secrets questionnaire, Tom discovered that his key word was Please, while Lisa's was Yes. Tom did not have a clear vision for their second birth, and discovered that on some level there was the feeling that he wanted to hand over responsibility for the birth to others. Yet, what lay beneath this was the desire to for a 'quick, efficient' labour.

Lisa did not feel that she was able to approach this birth with a strong sense of Yes due to her previous birth experience. She didn't feel safe enough to be able to let go and say Yes to birth, so we explored ways in which she could begin to feel safer and more trusting. This took Lisa to No, where she discovered that she needed to be clearer about her own truth. This meant going for the home birth she really wanted, but which she had not pursued because Tom was not supportive.

This took us back to Tom's 'vision' for birth, the vision of a 'quick, efficient labour' free from trauma. In discussing how to achieve this we looked at the physiology of birth and how an environment of privacy and trust best supported the release of important birthing hormones. Lisa would therefore benefit from being in the most relaxing environment for her so that she could surrender to the process without the fear or pressure of intervention. It was clear from this how it was possible to align both Tom and Lisa's needs and for them to move forward together.

Towards the end of her pregnancy Lisa revealed that she was feeling very vulnerable and asked if it was OK to be moving towards birth feeling 'uncoated' or emotionally exposed. This was the perfect place for Lisa to be, and indeed the softening hormone relaxin was contributing to these feelings. Exposing this level of vulnerability was new to Lisa, as it was to Tom – allowing themselves to be open and vulnerable with each other had brought a new dimension and closeness to their relationship. Tom, especially, was able to consider the idea that he did not need to rescue Lisa from her vulnerability, but that it was OK for him to simply meet and be with her in this place.

Their son was born at home on Boxing Day after a fast, efficient trauma-free labour. Lisa and Tom described how neither of them had realised how much they had needed to let go of the birth of their first child before they could really free the way for the birth of their second. They described this as a process of peeling or dropping away of layers. Lisa and Tom were able to come together to share the responsibility for the birth and work together in a mutually supportive way.

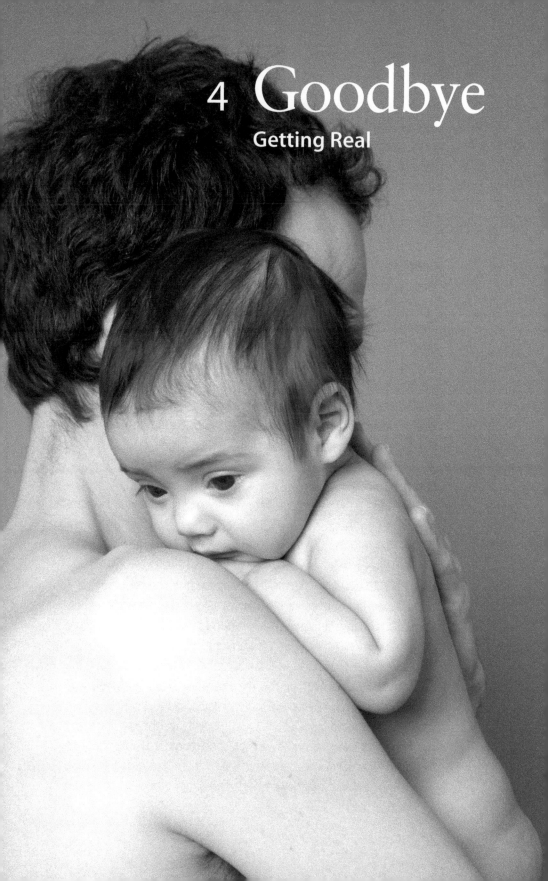

4 Goodbye

Getting Real

As we move forward on our pregnant journey with a stronger connection to our heart and a greater sense of appreciation nurtured by the state of Thank you, it's now time to face the magnitude of our passage into parenthood. This means it's time to wake up, make decisions and to let go of those things in our lives that will no longer be helpful to us if we are to fully embrace our responsibility as parents. Welcome to the fourth secret of a joyful birth: Goodbye.

Goodbye

Although it may feel challenging and uncomfortable (it takes us into new territory within ourselves, our relationships and the way in which we inhabit our body, and ask us to face our fears) the joy and freedom which it brings when we fully engage with what Goodbye demands of us is limitless. In pregnancy there is change on all fronts, yet when we face our fears and step courageously towards the next path that presents itself, we bring a grace and ease to each transition. In order to face our fears, however, we need to be truly awake to ourselves and to the decisions we are required to make.

Futures Collide

Discovering that we are pregnant is our first wake up moment: we are pregnant, from hereon in everything will change. Whether this is our first child or a further addition to the family, nothing will be the same again. Nevertheless, culturally, we tend to shy away from this reality. New parents, especially first time parents, are often asked if their life is back to normal yet even within a few weeks of the birth. But what is normal has changed. Life will never return to what was normal before this pregnancy.

Our first decision will be whether or not to sustain the pregnancy. For many of us this may be an obvious and welcome choice. For some, however, pregnancy may come as a shock and we may need time to decide what we want. Nevertheless, from the moment that we become aware of conception, it is important to recognise and acknowledge that there is an embryo growing inside our womb. Suddenly, we have more to think about than just ourselves, we have to make decisions for ourselves and the tiny life flowering within.

Walking The Line

If a pregnancy is welcomed and sustained, then we may exclaim: 'I am pregnant.' Immediately, we must accept and initiate change. Some changes may be small (attending to dietary needs, cutting down on caffeine and alcohol, getting more rest, for instance), others may be big (ending a relationship, making a life-long commitment to a relationship, moving house or reducing stress at work). Each of them will be about attending to the nitty-gritty of life and each of them is part of the process of expanding our perception of ourselves to include ourselves as a mother. With Goodbye we become more adult with each moment.

Letting Go

Every cycle comes to an end, and with every end there is a letting go. We have to let go of the past in order to make decisions. We then tie up loose ends and bravely move on. Pregnancy is a continual state of Goodbye. We even have a timescale and deadline for Goodbye: nine months, estimated due date. Then, with the birth of our baby one cycle ends and another begins.

So, we should ask: How do I cope with change? How do I do transitions? How do I approach the unknown? We need to be real about these questions, in order that we can be kind with and trusting of ourselves, gentle and honest with our partner, and so that we can seek the support and advice we need. Denial and inauthenticity are not helpful. Goodbye demands that we dive right in and attend to detail, we leave no stone unturned and we face up to our responsibilities.

Finding Ourselves

The responsibility of welcoming a new child into the world may mean that we start to make different choices about how we live and what we value. There may be a period of grief for the loss of life as we have known it, for the loss of space and time, and for the loss of the way we have previously enjoyed our relationship with our partner. It is not uncommon to hear a new mum say that she is scared that she is 'losing herself' in motherhood.

Inevitably, as we have said, there is that letting go of our old selves. But, within motherhood we will have the delight of exploring a new aspect of ourselves, and we can't even fathom what that might feel like until we are there, and even then it will continue to change and evolve. The only thing we can do, therefore, is to ready ourselves as best we can to be able to embrace these changes and allow ourselves the space and freedom to find ourselves where we are when we enter into motherhood with this child. Every child is unique and each can teach us new things about ourselves as women, as mothers, as parents.

One of the key aspects of our identity that we will come into a new relationship with is our career. When we go on maternity leave we have to let go of our job. This may be the first time in our lives when we have stepped out of our career, and all the ways in which we define our identity through our career. Maternity leave is not a holiday, a career break, or redundancy, it is an opportunity for us to be at home and to prepare for, and then enjoy, the next phase of our lives as mothers.

Understandably, this may herald a mixture of emotions. There may be relief at having more space to rest and relax as our growing body demands more from us. There may be relief at leaving behind the enormous pressure and stress that many people find at work. But, there may also be great sadness at leaving behind a role we loved doing, did well, received appreciation for, and saying goodbye to the colleagues we enjoyed working alongside.

It may feel frightening to hand over our role at work to someone else when we have no idea what our new role will be like at home. So, again, we come to the fundamental truth about Goodbye: we have to let go of one phase of our life without knowing what the future holds. We have to bold and trusting enough to take a leap of faith into the unknown. For some people this is easy. They are able to attend to the details that will allow them to step forward and move on. Many of us flounder though, we're not quite sure what we need to do, we struggle to be truthful and to let go.

Yet, embracing Goodbye means that we are able to birth more lightly. Birth is challenging enough for most women, we want to make it as easy for ourselves as possible. Meeting our responsibilities, facing our fears, letting go, moving on – all of this allows us to approach birth and parenting in a more relaxed way. In this way, we allow ourselves to be open to and to receive our baby with great joy.

Facing Fears

Every transition we make in life may carry with it an element of fear – fear of letting go of the past, fear of moving forward into the unknown. Many women experience fear and anxiety in pregnancy, not only in relation to childbirth, and particularly as we live in a culture that likes to fuel this fear, but also in relation to becoming a parent. How will we cope with our new responsibility, the responsibility of caring for and nurturing a new life? Who will we become in this role? Where will we find the strength we need to deal with the new challenges in our lives?

Often, where it is not apparent how we can fix fears, we tend to shy away from and refuse to acknowledge them. Yet, fears by their very nature are based on speculation and imagination, and so cannot always be fixed. However intangible fear may be though, it does have a tangible impact on our physiology. In birth, in the first stage of labour, fear can inhibit the flow of hormones such as oxytocin and endorphins, which are produced by the parasympathetic nervous system and which enable labour to progress and our body to produce its own pain relief. Fear produces the hormone adrenalin, which acts like a break for labour – contractions may slow, muscles may tighten and labour may come to a halt.

Rather than feeding our fears, therefore, we can choose to relax instead. Relaxation helps to dissipate fear and adrenalin, and encourages the release of the all-important hormones oxytocin and endorphins. If we can acknowledge our fears, then choose to relax, we are choosing a way forward that allows for letting go and release – which is exactly what we need to do on a physical level with our cervix, so that we can birth our baby.

Facing fears and then choosing to relax is not necessarily easy, though. It takes practise. Ideally, we practise this in our daily lives way before we even come to our birthing. Practising will help us enter and move through the state of Goodbye more gracefully, and indeed our fears are a good indicator of old patterns and emotions that we may need to say Goodbye to.

Naming our fears, in the presence of someone we trust and love, enables us to get real about what they are. It is important that our birth partner listens to our fears about birth. They do not need to fix our fears or to magic them away, but they do need to listen with kind intention and to ensure that we feel heard. If a birth partner can understand some of the fears a woman has been facing in her pregnancy, then they will be better able to respond to their needs in the birthing room.

So, now it's time to face some of your fears. Together with your birth partner, take a pen and paper, and each of you write down 1) three fears you have about the birth, and 2) three fears about the early postnatal period. Then, read aloud you fears to each other, in turn. Between you, do not attempt to solve, fix or belittle the fears. If you are listening, simply listen and state your partner's fear to show that you have heard them. Remember, fears are based on pure speculation, which are linked to past experiences, perhaps even unconscious ones. But, fears are not real – the mind has wandered into fearful territory, there is no reason to follow it.

If your fears have been heard in a respectful way, you may be able to hold them more lightly and recognise them for what they are. Waking up to yourself means waking up to all of yourself, not just the bits you like, but the bits that feel uncomfortable too. So, ask yourself which parts of you need attention? What do you need to wake up to? Be brave, dare to know yourself better.

Keywords

Entering the state of Goodbye might happen in a flash, an epiphany or eureka moment, or it might happen more gradually, we become aware that something is shifting within us and as it begins to dawn on us light is shed on those places that have become stuck within us. This aspect of Goodbye is realisation. The other three aspects associated with Goodbye may take much longer than realisation and we need to be prepared to run with the process in order to experience the joy and release of Goodbye. From realisation comes decision. Once we have made a decision there is the necessity to take action and follow through – this is completion. Once we have reached completion we can finally let go and move on.

Realisation

With the moment we discover our pregnancy comes realisation. Something has changed that has an immediate impact on our psyche, body and spirit. We now carry another human being within us and with that flows a river of different meanings that are unique to each individual. Our life is now in a very different place.

There may be a myriad of responses to pregnancy from joy and excitement to shock and dismay. While one woman says 'At last, how wonderful, I have waited so long,' another may say 'How terrible, this was not the plan, what shall I do?' Or we might sit somewhere in the middle: 'Great, I am pregnant. But, I would have preferred to get pregnant next year, not this month.' So, we need to be real with ourselves, face the truth of the moment, to challenge ourselves to be authentic so that we can embrace the next phase with more clarity.

While we can never assume what pregnancy means to another, we can assume that in some way each of us needs to wake up to the fact that decisions must now follow. To deny ourselves of this realisation, denies us the ability to make choices that are authentic and real for us in the given moment. Miss the moment and discomfort will follow – there will be that niggling feeling that says something needs to be acknowledged, that something has not been given the attention it deserves.

This niggling feeling is a constant reminder that we need to face what is happening, and what may follow – the need to realise that one phase of our lives has passed and another is beginning. If we don't get with this realisation then often the symptoms of change will get louder and louder until they are screaming for attention. 'Wake up', they yell, 'Notice me', they beg. We need to complete on the past, before we step into the future. If we shy away from this fact, then we may approach the new phase with a weightiness that may inhibit our ability to welcome the new phase with openness and freedom.

Nature articulately displays the cycles of death and rebirth, such is nature's law of constant change. Nature allows for the full completion and death in one cycle as it readies itself to be reborn. A tree easily lets go of its dead leaves before gathering its energy inwards for the winter and then sprouting fresh green shoots and leaves in the spring. Nature doesn't 'hold on' in the way humans can – we are creatures of habit and we like the familiar. Nature doesn't do denial. Denial does not serve life well.

We are either dying or growing all the time. In pregnancy we are both dying to who we were and growing into our new role. Avoiding realisation and fighting to keep oneself in the humdrum of familiarity are a kind of living death. We need to stay alive to change, to realise our new responsibilities and to be decisive.

Perineal Massage

The perineum is the tissue between your vagina and your anus. It stretches as your baby's head crowns in the opening of the vagina, allowing your baby to be born. Massaging your perineum has three main benefits: firstly, it helps you to get real about the fact that your baby is going to be born through your vagina. Secondly, since it is common to hold a lot of emotional tension in our pelvic region, it literally helps us to loosen up in readying for birth. Finally, perineal massage can help soften the tissue and prevent tearing.

Perineal massage can be done alone, or as a couple. Choose a time when you feel most relaxed, perhaps after a bath or as a prelude to lovemaking.

Massaging the perineal area during the last 3-4 weeks of pregnancy will help increase the elasticity of the tissues in this area and accustom you to the stretching sensations of second stage as the baby's head emerges. Perineal massage will not necessarily prevent a tear or the need for episiotomy, but it will help to increase stretchiness and de-sensitise the area to pressure and stretching.

Begin by lying back and using a mirror to locate the vagina and the perineum, between the vaginal opening and the anus. Using a natural vegetable oil on your thumbs, insert them 3-4cms inside the vagina and press the perineum towards the rectum and sides.

Gently stretch the opening until you feel a slight burning or tingling. Maintain pressure for 2 minutes until the area becomes a little numb. Then slowly massage in the oil, maintaining the stretch and pressure.

Massage for 3-4 minutes concentrating on any previous episiotomy scars which will be especially inelastic.

The massage can also be done with a sweeping motion from side to side, with the fingers either moving together in one direction or in opposite directions, according to your preference.

You can also get your partner to do this for you if you find it difficult to reach.

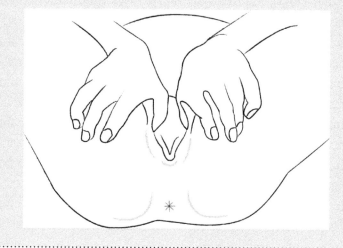

Decision

While trees easily let go of their leaves to move into the next phase of their lifecycle, we often hold onto old habits just in case. Yet, new skills are needed to meet the demands of this new stage of our lives, so we need to shed our old leaves and be open to receiving new ones, we need to decide what it is that will help us grow into motherhood. In this way, a Goodbye moment is bridge between the past and future.

In every Goodbye moment there is the opportunity to be mindful about how we choose to proceed. We are constantly presented with a chance to refine our decision making which, by turn, strengthens our identity. We are learning how to be less reactive, letting go of old patterns of behaviour, and more responsive, choosing to act in a way that is more about our essential truth than our conditioning. Truthful decisions are like feeding the roots of our being with a rich compost, through such decisions we nurture ourselves and allow ourselves to grow to our full potential.

So, as soon as we acknowledge our pregnancy we have decisions to make. Firstly, whether to continue with the pregnancy. That decided, then we have to consider lifestyle choices that will affect our growing baby. For instance, do we need to reduce our caffeine intake, steer clear of alcohol, eat healthier meals or get more rest? What other decisions need to be made to help us move forward?

Some people find decision so difficult they constantly totter in indecision. Others will wait until others make decisions for them, handing over their power to those whom they perceive 'know best'. This is irresponsible. We are adults and as adults we need to make decisions for ourselves. By avoiding such responsibility, we simply reinforce old patterns of behaviour, making them stronger and stronger, and harder and harder to let go of. It is better to realise as soon as possible that decisions need to be made and we have to make them. Of course, it is important to get input from other significant others in the baby's life, their father or co-parent, who will also be making their own decisions.

As humans we have free will. In order to exercise free will, we need to be fully open ourselves and to engage with the depths of our being. This means we need to look inside ourselves, not outside. The actions we take as a consequence of our decisions give form to our inner workings – our actions show that we have clearly met and are responding to our responsibilities. It is crucial, therefore, that we make authentic decisions that support who we are. Sometimes, though, it can be difficult to connect with our sense of Self. In this case, it is helpful to think about decisions we made in the past and reflect on those which were supportive and nurturing, and those which were less so. What can we learn from past processes?

This does not, however, mean that we are looking for the easiest choice or decision. The best decision is not always the most comfortable one. For instance, if a woman is in a violent relationship and discovers she is pregnant, she may decide to keep the baby but maybe challenged to get real about the state of her relationship and how that may impact the baby. Any decision to leave the relationship maybe extremely difficult in the short term, but incredibly nourishing in the long term, for her and for her baby.

Being aware of what happened around conception may tell us something about the way we do Goodbye. For some it may be a thought-out and conscious conception, for others it may be that the condom wasn't to hand and lust took over. Or, it could be that the baby was conceived even though contraception was used. Each individual set of circumstances will colour the ground upon which decisions will follow. So, again we must be careful to make decisions that are responsive, not reactive. It is no use burying our heads in the sand. If this is the case, we may need to reflect back to the first secret of a joyful birth, No, which is about creating a clear identity and establishing boundaries that help us to make authentic decisions that best reflect our truth.

There are two aspects of decision making: head and heart, and the two are not necessarily opposing. Our decisions need to be based on informed choices, we need to do our research and engage our thinking brain. But, they also need to be based on intuition. When we lay all the information and advice to one side for a few moments, and sit peacefully with ourselves, which decision feels 'right'? In this way we bring together our understanding of what we observe in the outer world and what, internally, we feel is the right path for us and our baby.

Since decisions also speak of commitment, each one must be in alignment with who we are and support our personal identity, for how can we act and complete on something if we do not wholeheartedly agree with it? Yet, in pregnancy, we do also need to co-operate with our baby and partner so that we make decisions which reflect the good of all. This may bring with it the realisation that we are in a relationship with someone who has different values to us – or a realisation for our partner in this way. For example, while a couple may feel they agree on most things, when it comes to birth there might be quite different belief systems at play. The woman may feel she wants a normal home birth, while the father may have grown up in a household where birth was regarded as dangerous and homebirth is considered an act of selfishness on the woman's part. In such instances, the couple will have to realise their differences before they can come together to make a joint decision that accurately reflects the path they wish to take.

Clearly, then, where parenting touches on our own experiences of being parented, it can bring about huge differences of opinion when we consider decisions that will directly affect our child – birth, vaccination, early years care, and schooling are but a few of the major decisions we will have to face and find our own way through as a family.

Whereas choices are about exploring personal preferences, decisions cut deeper and demand commitment. Decisions are not to do with right or wrong, rather the way in which we express the truth of who we are as parents. Once we have made a decision, we affirm the course of life that flows from it, putting other distractions aside. A decision is resolute, it brings clarity and making it known to others can cement it further, allowing them to rally round to support us in our commitment. Pregnancy is not a time to hide around decision-making. The world celebrates any movement towards truth and wakefulness, and being open to receive that may make it easier for us to make and complete on the decisions we take.

Completion

While realisation may happen in an instant and decision over a relatively short period of time, the next aspect of Goodbye – completion – may take much longer. It demands time and energy to finish what we have started, and involves an act of will that will bring with it a sense of dignity and the satisfaction and joy of seeing something through. We all need to learn this skill, the ability to do whatever is needed in order to complete, however boring it may get along the way – it is all too easy to become distracted by the new and move quickly onto new projects and thoughts of the future that feel more exciting.

Making a decision may not always be enough to move forwards, though; we need to deal with the sticky strands of the past before we can fully embrace the next stage of our lives. In birth, for instance, a couple may be excited by the decision to go for as natural and straight-forward a birth as possible. This decision is merely the beginning of a process that will require commitment and work to follow through, including gathering information, examining our beliefs around birth, talking to midwives and antenatal teachers about what will be most helpful in this journey, and finding the right kind of support. It also involves putting to rest those attitudes, beliefs, relationships, and so on, that will not be helpful to us on this path. Completion is the action that makes a decision come into being.

Completion often asks us to strengthen our boundaries, our No, so that we can let go of those things we have realised will get in the way of us moving on. In terms of social life, for instance, a couple may decide that they need to make a change in their lifestyle from going out a lot to staying in more and taking time to rest and prepare for birth and parenting. They may then need to be more boundaried with friends who expect them to go out and party and continue to live their lives in the same way.

That's not to say that there won't be differences between a pregnant woman and her partner. A degree of negotiation may be essential. For instance, a pregnant woman may expect her partner to give up alcohol, but her partner may not want to or feel they need to.

But it is important that such nitty-gritty is attended to, so that both partners can move forwards freely into the next stage of the journey.

In this way, completion may bring about 'now or never' feelings – it's now or never that we clean up our lifestyle for the good of the baby. Reducing stress at work, for instance, is something that we may keep putting off, but if we are to thrive in pregnancy and enter birth and parenting in a more relaxed state, then it calls for immediate action. Again, such challenges are not always easy to find our way through. It can be painful and may cause conflict when we tell our colleagues and our partner that certain practices or behaviours have to change if we are to get our pregnant needs met.

Goodbye, then, is not for the conflict-adverse – though with a clear No, we do not need to approach it in an aggressive, proud or defensive way. Family and friends do get used to us acting in a certain way, however, so initially they may be very resistant to change. But, if we can stand back a little and choose to observe reactions from a more detached point of view, then we will see that this resistance simply highlights where people are stuck and what it brings up for them to see others moving forward in their lives.

Indeed, emotions are often what get in the way of a clean completion. We can notice and feel our emotions, but then choose not to let them rule our decisions. If we swing from one emotion to another and make decisions based on their inconsistent nature, then we risk moving into the next phase of our lives carrying emotional baggage that keeps pulling us back into old and unhelpful habits. None of this is going to happen quickly, settling our affairs takes time, but it is part of our responsibility as expectant parents. Pregnancy is a time to grow up, to see where we have previously struggled in our lives, and to bring attention to what needs to be done to change those patterns and help us to feel more liberated in the future. Ultimately, no-one else can birth our baby, and no-one else is responsible for those things that get in the way of us doing so freely, from a place of clarity, love and joy.

Sometimes it can be easier to see the process of completion playing out in our career, than in our personal lives, though. A pregnant woman must hand over her responsibilities at work to a colleague or new recruit before she goes on maternity leave. This involves tying up all sorts of loose ends and may involve painful emotions. It is not always easy to hand over something you have worked so hard for to someone else, and to accept that they can do the job just as competently, albeit differently, as you. Refusing to complete and carrying work over into maternity leave, may be a way of holding onto our old lives rather than embracing the new. Surrendering and letting go can leave us feeling vulnerable and uneasy, and so it is no wonder that we like to feel like we will always be in control.

Waking Up To Your Pregnancy

Give yourself time to consider the following questions in a quiet place where there is no likelihood of distractions. If you are in a couple, invite your partner to answer the relevant questions too. Allow yourself to be open and honest with all that comes forward, letting your baby know these are your thoughts and emotions and that they are not to be taken on in anyway them.

- How do you feel about your pregnancy?
- How do you feel about your changing body?
- As a partner, how do you feel about this pregnancy?
- As a partner, how do you feel about your pregnant partner's changing body?
- What impact does each of you feel this baby will have on your relationship?
- What decisions could you make and complete on in order to support your couple relationship, so that together you are able to grow into this transition?
- How do you feel about the birth and each stage of labour – stage one is dilation of the cervix, stage two is pushing and birth of the baby, stage three is the birth of the placenta, stage four is bonding and feeding?

- What decisions could you make and complete on that would help you to support each other through this process? Individually, what do you need to do to prepare for birth?
- How does each of you feel about becoming a parent?
- What decisions could you make and complete on to support your transition into parenthood?
- What now needs to happen differently to make this transition feel as comfortable as possible? For instance, what changes do you need to make to your lifestyle? What emotional support do you need? Where can you make time to nurture each other? Where can you make time to give each their own space? Where can you find positive role-models for parenting, and how can you spend more time with these people?
- How do your families of origin embrace any changes that you make to the way you live your life? Do you resonate with their response? Do you need to create some boundaries that will allow your new family to grow and develop in the way you would like it to?

Moving On

Every day, every moment of our lives, we are moving on and the final moving on comes with death. To resist this premise, is to resist life itself. Life changes, that is its only constant. We will associate with different people at different times in our life. Some may travel a long way with us, our lovers, partners, family, children; others may only be with us for a few months or years. But, ultimately we move onto the next world alone.

When we feel the depth of one chapter closing and another beginning, it can bring a great sense of intimacy and sweetness to life. There can also be clarity and purpose when we feel that we are in alignment with the flow of our lives. If we have, truthfully, followed

92

through the process of realisation, decision and completion then it will be easier to move on toward birth and parenting with ease and grace. But, if we continue to ignore those loose ends and shirk our responsibilities, then moving on will be experienced in a very different way. It may feel gross, burdensome, difficult.

It is the heart's knowing that carries us forward and enables us to embrace each new phase. Sadness may be part of this process. For instance, a pregnant woman may miss the lightness of her pre-pregnant body, while at the end of her pregnancy she may grieve her pregnant body once she has given birth. This does not mean she is not happy to be pregnant or that she does not love her newborn baby. With each step forward there is a moving on and letting go of the past, and we should acknowledge all the emotions that arise along the way.

Recognising that loss is an aspect of any Goodbye moment is vital; it helps us to be real about where we are, and makes it easier to move on. Allowing old issues, feelings and emotions to show themselves and pragmatically dealing with them as they arise, releases energy and vitality. In this way, there is a great power to moving on since the world reaches out to support us. We need to stay open to what comes forward during this process – unless we deal with things as they arise, the obstacles will become bigger and bigger until we finally get real and deal with the underlying issues. Just like emotions, obstacles can disappear as quickly as they appeared if we acknowledge them, attend to them and allow ourselves to move on. During pregnancy our wake up calls or Goodbye moments are an opportunity to clear up the mess, to cut a path through the undergrowth and to walk our way to freedom in our birth and parenting. But, this takes courage and tenacity, and there's certainly no place for sleeping in denial. So, wake up to joy.

Accepting Loss

Often Western culture hides away from the shadowy sides of human experience. And, especially in pregnancy, we might feel that we should be happy all the time. But, this is not real. Indeed, for us to experience more joy in our birth and parenting, as in our lives, it is vital that we embrace all the different shades and colours of our experience. Pregnancy, birth and parenting may bring up sadness and grief, and we need to let ourselves be open to feeling such emotions. Every change, every step away from the old towards the new, carries with it an element of loss. So, be honest with yourself and explore your feelings around your pregnancy in an open and non-judgmental way. This is part of being kind to yourself during this time.

Do you feel any degree of sadness or fear within yourself at this time? Where does this sadness or fear originate, where is it focused? Changes in your body and perception of yourself? Around relationship changes? Work changes? How easily can you accept that one phase of your life is ending, and another is beginning? What is this change asking of you – what do you need to let go of in order to make space for the new? Would it be helpful to take another look at your No (see chapter one), so that you can develop a stronger connection with what is truthful for you in your birth and parenting?

Does the timing of this pregnancy feel right? Do you feel that you are in flow with your life? What do you need to wake up to be fully present to this journey, fully present for this precious new life growing within? What do you need to do in order to align yourself with this pregnant journey?

Do you feel the time-liness of this pregnancy? Do you feel in the flow of your life? Can you get the call to wake up and show up for this precious journey as you nurture the growth of a new life? What do you need to do to align yourself with this pregnant journey?

Hello Baby!

Culturally there can often be a disconnection between a woman's pregnancy and a very real acknowledgment of the baby growing within. While many people understand the biology, the division of cells, the development of those cells into a foetus which will then be born as a baby, it may be harder for them to conceive of baby as having their own experiences, their own feelings and emotions. But, babies in utero are people, they are intelligent, sentient beings and it is important that they are recognised as such from the outset. Some women may even have a connection with their baby before it is conceived and there is increasing scientific evidence to show that babies have an experience that involves memory in utero, that the mind exists even before there is any brain matter. So, wake up. There is another being here with you, now. How does it feel to acknowledge that your baby is having experiences all the time, which will have an impact on the way in which it develops?

Babies' experiences in utero lay down all kinds of foundations for their future, including the foundations of a healthy nervous system. While a moderate amount of stress during pregnancy has been shown to improve motor and mental development in a young child, if a baby experiences high levels of stress during pregnancy consistently there may be a whole range of implications for that baby which may extend into their adulthood. If a baby is flooded by stress hormones from its mother during its time in the womb, then they may experience the embodiment process as more stressful. In other words, that becoming a human being is a stressful experience.

Yet, acknowledging this is not about creating a raft of guilt for mothers. Rather, it is about waking up to the fact that your experiences may impact your baby's experience, whether that's stress, relaxation, nourishing food, and enjoying such pleasures as good company and music that touch you on a soul level. So, with this new awareness, would it be possible for you to make a commitment to regularly gift your baby with the art of relaxation, so that at least for some part of each day they experience a cocktail of relaxation hormones?

If, however, the reality is that life is stressful for you at present, or at any point in your pregnancy, you can honour your baby by owning your experience. It's as simple as talking to them: 'Sorry that you are experiencing stress hormones at the moment. This stress is mine, not yours, and I am doing all I can to take care of it.' In this way, you validate your baby's experience.

Such communication need not be confined to pregnancy. When a baby shows signs of distress in labour, then it can be helpful to talk to baby and encourage them to relax, even though the experience of labour may feel very strong and challenging – even natural, straightforward labour maybe full on for baby, this is a completely new experience for them just as each labour is a completely new experience for mum. Time after time, I have heard couples describe how talking to the baby has helped to lessen the distress and to relax baby enough to bring their heart rate back down to a normal level.

Staying present to your baby's experience is one of the decisions you can make that will help you to work with the realisation that your baby and your journey is unique, that by establishing connection with baby and validating their experience early on you are laying strong foundations for their health and their experience of relationship for years to come. Your contact will help reassure them through every experience, including those such as birth which may be frightening for both of you.

Not for all, but for the vast majority, women experience labour as more powerful and demanding than any other experience they have ever had. So accept that, prepare your mind as well as your body, and give yourself time so that you can approach it in as relaxed and resourced a way as possible. In many cultures, if you were about to embark on a special journey that would change you forever, some kind of rite of passage, there would be ceremony and ritual designed to initiate and prepare you. But, these days, you may need to be your own wise woman, to be your own warrior. So, be prepared for yourself, and be prepared for your baby.

Case Study 4: *Sorry, Goodbye*

Sarah

Sarah was 30 weeks pregnant when we did the Seven Secrets questionnaire. She was an older mum who had ridden a long and active path to pregnancy involving four IVF cycles and much energy and attention put towards working with body-mind healing. She had actually got pregnant after attending a retreat in the USA where she had had a major release and suddenly knew that pregnancy would follow (it did) after ten years of attempting conception. This was a very wanted baby.

It was in the state of Sorry that the questionnaire took us. Sarah was having a tussle between what being responsible meant. She described it as a struggle between the body versus logic. What was "the most responsible" way to approach the birth. When we explored this deeper Sarah talked about having a very negative and critical mothering experience herself, and how this left her with a tendency to be very hard on herself. Her mother had always had a fearful approach to pregnancy and Sarah felt could see the need to protect herself from this attitude at this time. Sarah felt she was having to balance her desire for a natural birth with the knowledge that if help was needed then she wanted to be ready to accept that help. She didn't want to go through a long labour and end with an emergency section.

Most of the exploring that we did focused on Sarah and her experience of mothering, especially at that time of puberty when a young girl is transitioning to adulthood. She said what came forward for her when she considered this time of her life, was that when she was 14 she had had an ovarian cyst the size of a football which meant she menstruated for six months. She told no-one at the time though eventually her mum noticed it. We could really acknowledge the 14 year old Sarah who had felt so alone and "wrong" at that time. She took on a feeling that she had to be hard on herself, especially in the area of female fertility, added to by her mum's negative attitude to children.

We ended the session with Sarah taking responsibility for herself in a way that didn't mean she was going to burden herself with "having to get it right". Having seen some of the family patterning around birth and parenting enabled Sarah to step forward more freely, realizing that she could only do her best whatever that was. This took some of the pressure away from Sarah in terms of having to approach the birth in such a "loaded" way. She didn't feel that she was going to scrutinize her every move in the same judgmental way. She was also willing to be open to the form of her birth rather than have a fixed picture she had to adhere to which wouldn't allow her freedom to go with the flow. There were some considerations that meant she was being called to approach the birth with an open mind.

Sarah gave birth to a beautiful baby boy by caesarean birth. Early on in the labour as progress was slow and baby was showing some signs of stress Sarah made the decision with her husband that they didn't want to wait and see if baby would get more distressed, but take decisive action now. She felt very accepting that for her, with her long and involved journey in getting pregnant, that this was the way that felt most ok. She didn't feel the need to pressurize herself but rather accepted that the way they chose to go was right for them and the start of their family. She felt able to meet her baby with undiluted joy and excitement.

Interestingly the state of Sorry was there to be revisited after birth in that there was an awareness of her mum and her attitude potentially affecting the postnatal field. Her mum had never been maternal and even then stated "I can't see why you wanted one". Sarah wanted to stay in a place where she healed and nurtured her relationship with her mum, involving her in her new grandson's life. She chose to "look through" appearances and trust that actually her mum's words didn't convey the whole story. In this way she nurtured a blossoming relationship between grandmother and grandson, and would on many occasions catch her mother talking to her grandson in such an affectionate and warm way that even at her mum's stage of life (she is in her 80s) there was room for change in perceptions around children. If Sarah hadn't been so committed to healing the sadness in herself around receiving the negative attitudes around parenting, she may not have been able to be so open to her mother's humanness and wounding. The state of Sorry is a journey into accepting our humanness and that of others, faults and all.

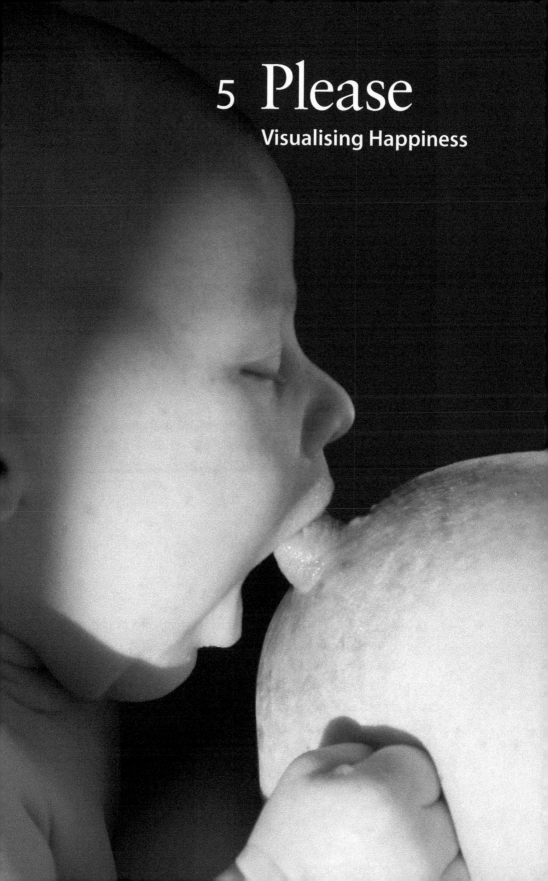

5 Please

Visualising Happiness

How many of us have a vision of what we want from our lives? And, how many of us know how to ask for what we need to make that happen? What would we have to do to believe that if we were to ask for something, we would get it? This is secret five of a joyful birth: Please.

Please

In order to acknowledge what we don't want in our lives, we have to confront our fears about change – Goodbye (chapter four). Sometimes it may also be difficult to see the opportunities that are in front of us – Hello (chapter two). At other times we might be inhibited by a lack of self-worth – a dysfunctional Thank you (chapter three). What usually happens is that we tend to get stuck in a loop, going round in circles, again and again, producing the same results. Indeed, it's a classic self-help adage that if you always do what you've always done, you'll always get what you've always got.

Yet, when we connect with our No, Hello, Thank you and Goodbye in an authentic way, then we begin to realise the huge potential of Please. Rather than remaining stuck in that loop, Please breaks the cycle and opens the way to another path, along which we will discover every kind of opportunity. The circular pattern then begins to spiral outwards, which has a completely different form and momentum and which represents a progression towards a higher goal, towards a refinement of our being.

Focus, Please

Once we accept our inner authority, which we can find by exploring No (chapter one), we can then be confident about asking for and getting what we want. Please demands that we have a clear vision of what we want, the intention to put into action those things that will helps us achieve our goal(s), and an awareness of the need for cooperation with others to help us get there. Finally, we need to bring a spiritual quality to our vision and it is through prayer that we reach out to and ask for help from a higher being, whether we choose that being to be God, Love or some other form that resonates with our personal spiritual beliefs.

All of this requires focus and commitment. By freeing ourselves from old patterns and creating a new vision for our lives, we are changing our position in the world, which will inevitably affect others around us. If we can be strong in this, and invite others to change too, then we will become stronger in ourselves, shifting and shaping the course of many people's lives, not least our own, our partner's and our baby's. Yet, in doing this, we must tread a path of modesty and humility, and we must also be prepared to take absolute responsibility for ourselves and for everything that we ask.

The Please Of Birth

Only when we have a clear vision for our birth and parenting are we ready to begin the journey. Without clear vision, we are in danger of bumbling along with little sense of where we are going, wandering, getting lost and wasting energy. A lack of vision will also make it difficult to get the support we need. After all, if we don't know what we want, how can we ask others to help us along the way?

Getting clear about what we want starts at the moment of conception, and is all about communication. There are two people involved in conception, so that means both people in the relationship need to nurture their own vision and then come together to agree a way forward. It is all too easy to assume, based on our own experiences, that we know what the other person wants without ever asking them – and listening to – what it is they need. We might complain that our partner doesn't meet our needs, criticising them for where we perceive them to be lacking. But, how often are we really clear about what we need? And how clearly do we then communicate that to our partner?

The timing has to be right for both partners to be able to think about and then explain what they want. Each partner will need to explore such questions as family set-up (including professional work, managing the home, childcare, housing, and so on) and birth preferences (hospital birth, home birth, NHS versus an independent midwife, doula, medical pain relief, self-help pain relief, etc.). Each must be given the space to offer their opinion and reflect on the choices that are right for them. It is then time to come together to agree what needs to happen next.

Coming Together

When we come together as a couple to work towards a vision of our birthing and parenting then we will feel stronger and more confident. Consequently, everything will start to flow more easily. Birthing is a huge event in a woman's , man's and a baby's life, and we need to be fully supported on that journey. Cooperation between the pregnant woman and her partner will benefit everyone and create strong foundations for the parenting that follows.

A joint vision must meet the needs of mother, father/parent and baby, and will highlight where other sources of support is required. What is key, though, is to define the essence of the vision. So, what is at heart of our birthing? We might hope for a peaceful home birth with a water pool and no intervention, but what if, during our birthing the form of the birth changes? What if we need to transfer to hospital? What if we need drugs to cope with the intensity of contractions caused by the use of synthetic hormones that speed up the progress of labour? What if there is a need for an intrumental delivery with ventouse or forceps, or a caesarean section?

Such elements as making informed decisions, staying actively engaged in the process so that we understand our options at each turn of events, hiring a doula to provide extra emotional and practical support, and acknowledging and validating the baby's experience throughout are all fundamental choices that will support the underlying sacredness of our vision for birth. A vague vision statement such as 'a natural home birth, please,' will not serve us well if things don't go to plan. Ultimately, we cannot predict what will happen in our birthing. It is one of the biggest steps into the unknown that we can take.

Keywords

Vision, intention, cooperation and prayer. Each of these four aspects of Please are equal, though some are perhaps more equal than others. While we may have a clear idea of what we want (vision) and ask the world, universe, God, whatever we like to call it, to help us achieve our goals (prayer), neither of these is of any consequence without intention and cooperation. Intention is the action, energy and effort, required to

102

make things happen; cooperation is asking for and valuing the support and advice of others who can help us along the way. So, if we want to have a positive, empowering experience of birth, whatever our birth may look like, then the question is how much energy are we really prepared to invest in our vision in order to make it a reality?

Vision

Vision is the state in which we can allow ourselves to believe that anything and everything is possible. It provides all the answers to such questions as: 'What if I could have anything/do anything/be anything… I wanted, how would that look? What would it feel like?' Vision calls forth the imaginings of the heart and then invites us to find solutions and creative ways in which to make the possible possible.

A wonderful part of the process of preparing for birth and parenting is to give ourselves permission to freely envision our ideal pregnancy, birth and parenting. It frees up the psyche to work without restraint, dissolving negative patterns and bringing forward news ways of being. It is an immensely enjoyable and responsible way to meet pregnancy, as it asks us to engage with and shape the beginning of the journey with our child. It sharpens our ability to make good and truthful choices, and creates a map which we can refer to at any point. Until we take time to envision our birthing, it may not be clear what it is we actually value. We might be so locked in negative patterns of fear and anxiety that we don't even give ourselves the chance to make up our own minds about this journey. We should remind ourselves, frequently: 'This is my pregnancy, my birth, my child. So what choices would I like to make?'

Asking ourselves these questions enables us to get grounded in our ideas, to notice where we are being vague and to get clear about what we want. This is most certainly worth giving time and attention. So, what if we suspended any disbelief and gave ourselves a paintbrush to paint our ideal picture of birth? We can let the paintbrush go in any direction it likes and be open to what is revealed. In doing so, we resist the influence of peers, family, friends and instead be completely honest with ourselves. For instance, we may be surrounded by women who are opting for home births and we might assume that we would like the same. However, in our visioning we might discover that we would prefer to birth in a birth centre or hospital. If we can't allow ourselves to explore all the options, we might start to make choices that are not truthful for us.

Vision is not about fluffy daydreams in which everything is pink and sweet and nice, though. Fantasy alone does not stand up to the rigours of the living world. A realisable vision is one in which we align ourselves with our individual principles and purposes and act from our own unique spirit. True vision is the gift of heroes and heroines, the stuff of myth and timeless truths. This takes work and courage, and it is a challenge that most of us will find, well, challenging.

If we can cast aside the roles that have been set out for us by others and awaken to the hero/ine within, we can step out of other people's visions, step away from pressures of fears that inhibit our freedom, and thereby connect with our soul's purpose. Goodbye is the grounding for this. If we can master the qualities of the fourth secret of a joyful birth – realisation, decision, completion, moving on – then we may feel confident enough to go forward. When we refuse to feel fearful about change, we are then able to envision more freely, to see the bigger picture and to understand the depth of what is unfolding.

Pregnancy might be the first time we have allowed ourselves to be architects of our own future. For some women, the responsibility of carrying another being gives them the ability to shape their lives in way they have not done so before. This is why so many women find pregnancy, birthing and motherhood to be empowering and freeing rather than restricting.

So, we need to wake up to the heroine within. Perhaps it is time to ask for a helpful guide or mentor – a friend, doula, midwife, antenatal teacher – who can inspire us to step outside our habitual ways of thinking. This reminds us of the second secret of a joyful birth, Hello, which asks us to be open to what is around us. The sharper our vision, the greater the likelihood that we will find just the right person to help us when we need them.

What's important, however, is to understand that vision is not ambition. Ambition is quite different. For instance, if we over-focus on goals and become inflexible, then we are in danger of getting stuck in old patterns. Being goal-oriented about the form of our birth is not helpful. Setting ourselves up for a pass or fail completely misses the point. What is infinitely more helpful, however, is being truthful about what is at the heart of our vision for birth and being open to and accepting of the journey. This has nothing to do with ego and everything to do with the expression of the soul. We have nothing to prove and plenty to be joyful about.

Creating A Vision Of Birth

When creating your vision of birth, let your imagination be free to roam as it pleases. Don't let fear inhibit your flow and, similarly, don't let other people's expectations sabotage the process. You are in charge here, you make the decisions, you create your own set of values. If you wish to do this exercise as a couple, then each write your own list before coming together to listen to each other's vision and then creating a joint vision. In the joint vision, you might want to give baby some say in the matter too – what do you think baby would like to see in the vision, a vision that supports all three of you?

In creating a vision, you may find it helpful to work through each of the Seven Secrets of a Joyful Birth, jotting down your thoughts and ideas as you go. Give yourself as much time as you need. It is not necessary for you to have read chapters six (Sorry) or seven (Yes) to complete this exercise, though you might find it helpful to refer back to your vision once you have read them.

1. What is the NO of your birthing? What do you not want for your birth? Remember here that establishing clear boundaries helps to strengthen your identity, which will then make it easier to make decisions that reflect your truth.

2. What is the HELLO of your birthing? Where are you putting your attention? Are you open to new ideas? Are you able to exchange freely with others? Do you feel able to commune with baby in a relaxed, open way? What support would you need to be able to do this?

3. What is the THANK YOU of your birthing? Can you relax into a relationship of giving and receive with your baby? (Baby gives in many ways – for instance, sharing its life with you and being open to you as parent – and baby receives all kinds of things from you, such as attention, food, a safe place in which to grow and come into human form.) How do you appreciate your pregnancy? Your birthing? Your baby? Your partner? What helps you feel good inside, full of heart and love?

4. What is the GOODBYE of your birthing? What realisations have you had (about pregnancy, birthing, parenting, yourself and so on) and have you made decisions that support those realisations? Are you able to complete on those decisions? What supports you in this process of moving on? What helps you release fear?

5. What is the PLEASE of your birthing? What would your birth look like if you took away all fears, anxieties and limitations? Who would be there to help you? What would your ideal birthing environment look and feel like? How can you ask for the cooperation of others? Can you make time for moments of stillness in your life in which to offer up a prayer of your vision?

6. What is the SORRY of your birthing? What issues do you need to resolve so that they don't get in the way of your birth? Is there an area in your life for which you do not take responsibility? Are there any relationships that need to be repaired so that you can feel more peaceful within yourself? What guilt or self-judgment are you carrying around with you that might inhibit your birthing? What would help you release these feelings?

7. What is the YES of your birthing? What would you need to do/feel in order to be able to surrender to the process? How will you nurture your spiritual side in your birthing? How easily will you be able to find acceptance within yourself, whatever your birth looks like?

Intention

So how is a vision different from a wish? Well, a vision demands that we have the will to make it happen. It is something we want, so we will engage with whatever or whomever we need to in order to make it real. Often this means we need to go public with our vision, and this takes courage as it opens us to judgement from others. Commonly, we may be fearful that people will question our right to our vision, provoking such comments as, 'Who do you think you are?' If we say we would like a relaxed and orgasmic birth, then others may sneer and ask why we think we're so special that we can have or achieve such a birth. Sticking to our guns, holding our vision sacred in our own hands, as usual, requires commitment, effort and energy.

The arrow that takes us to the target of our vision, therefore, is intention. Without will or intention we will fall short of the mark. Often we will need to do some target practice every day to ensure a bulls eye when it comes to our birthing or parenting. Target practice might include practising relaxation and repeating positive affirmations daily, acquiring new skills and understanding through weekly antenatal classes, or asking those around us with positive ideas about and experiences of birth to be our mentor. A mentor could be a friend who demonstrates the qualities which are important for us in our vision, an experienced independent midwife, or a kind and attentive doula.

When we hold a clear vision in our mind's eye, we can question every step that we take. Why are we doing this? Does it serve our vision? In this way we will more easily align our action(s) with our vision, ensuring that we are on the right path. When we question our actions in this way, it becomes clear how habits and behaviour patterns can send us way off the mark. We can see more clearly when old fears and anxieties are getting in our way, and hopefully we can then discover what it is we need to do to find a way through and stay on this new path. We need to give ourselves time to do this, to give ourselves enough space in our lives be more mindful. Everything we do from the company we keep, the ways we spend our free time, the food we eat, what we read, what we watch on TV, and more, will all be either supporting and strengthening our vision, or undermining it. So, we need to get clear, stay real and be 100 per cent truthful with ourselves.

When we act from a place of true vision and intention, it brings a feeling of joy and excitement that comes from deep within. So, when we make choices, it is a good idea to check how each decision feels in our body. Do we feel uplifted? Do we feel energised? We let our body, with its connection to these feelings of lightness and freedom, be the judge. It is fine to indulge in the sensuous realms of desire and fantasy, but when making decisions we need to be disciplined enough to keep our vision and sense of higher purpose in mind.

Birth Preferences

In preparing for birth, you may be asked to draw up a birth 'plan'. But, what happens if your birth doesn't go according to plan? For this reason, I'd rather encourage you to put together a list of your birth 'preferences', to which you and your carers can refer to, but which also allows for flexibility, change and acceptance in your birthing. Birth preferences give those attending your birth a clearer insight into you as a person, and what you hold important in your birthing. The more people understand where you're coming from, the better the support they will be able to give you.

So, once you have created your vision of birth (see above), you may then like to use the following as a checklist for your birth preferences. This should be clear and easy to read, so that you can talk about it with your partner, midwife or consultant and doula, where appropriate. The list below is not comprehensive, so you may want to include other things that spring to mind, or that you discover as you research your birthing options.

- Where would you like to birth?
- Who would you like at your birth?
- What would you like to do during the early stages of labour?
- What would you like to eat and drink?

- Would you like to listen to music? If so, what?
- What kind of atmosphere do you want in the birthing room?
- What do you need to help you cope with pain?
- Would you like a water birth?
- What would you like to do during the second stage of labour?
- Would you like to see your baby's head crowning?
- Would you like your baby delivered directly onto you?
- Do you want to wait until the umbilical cord stops pulsating before it is cut?
- Do you want your baby to be cleaned before you have skin to skin?
- Do you want your baby to be examined immediately after birth or to wait for an hour before this happens?
- Do you want to breastfeed?
- Would you like to try for a physiological (natural) third stage?
- Would you like your midwife to show you your placenta?
- Would you like to keep your placenta?
- Do you want your baby to have Vitamin K? Injection? Or orally?
- What visitors, if any, do you want in the first few hours and days?

Cooperation

It is very hard to realise any kind of vision without the help of others. This can be very humbling, but it can also be a huge source of relief. It may feel infinitely safer for us to do things alone if we have been living in this way, yet vision requires that we integrate our intention with the intention of others to realise a higher purpose. In this way we will feel more powerful, more supported and more resourced in our journey towards a joyful birth. It gives width and depth to our vision, and allows us to shine more brightly.

Each individual needs to pull together, this means that each partner in a couple needs to cooperate with the other and believe in the vision of their birth or parenting. Cooperating in this way may be a challenge in itself for a couple. Yet, when both partners are aligned in a vision that furthermore acknowledges and validates the baby's experience they can work as a phenomenal team.

In cooperating with others we may need to revaluate our self-perceptions, or exercise compromise. In birth, compromises around pain relief may need to be made for instance. If a woman is clear that she wants to use medical pain relief but is also clear that she also wants the birth to be a positive experience for the baby, then she may decide to use drugs that least effect the baby. This will require research into the different effects of available drugs on the baby, and/or she might decide to consider other things such as a birthing pool and a doula that will strengthen her ability to cope with pain naturally.

In Western culture, we tend to celebrate individuality in a way that can keep us separate from others and we can often feel that we need to defend or hold onto a position that we deem to be right. While it is necessary to acknowledge and accept one's individual preferences, by clinging to our own individuality too strongly we run the risk of being blind to the bigger picture. So, especially when we hit a dead end or face an uncomfortable challenge, it is important not to separate ourselves from the support that will bring us back into alignment with our vision and allow us to feel a greater connection to the whole. Birth is a sum of parts – baby, mother, father/partner. Each needs to work cooperatively as best they can and be open to receiving support from each other.

As I have said, it is important for both partners in the couple to first create their own vision before coming together to form a joint vision. Each person can then feel heard and valued, and a sense of inter-connectedness will then follow. When we share our vision in this way we are allowing some part of our soul to be seen more clearly. This is part of the magic of embodiment. We reveal our hopes and aspirations to the world, and so bring them closer to form. Amazingly, we may be understood by those around us in a way we had not been before – and, similarly, we may see those around is a way that we had not previously done.

Cooperation illuminates certain qualities of human relationship such as empathy, understanding and acceptance. It enables us to start to experience the truth that our joy really is another's joy, and vice versa. We can let go of our attachment to self-service, and begin to discover the deep joy in serving another. This is a wonderful place to be at the beginning of our parenting journey, since parenting is founded on unconditional love and the ability to see and be open to what another person needs.

There is a fine balance, however, between personal vision and cooperation. We should not lose sight of our personal vision. Whenever we notice that we are moving too far away from our own truth as we join with others, then we need to realise that it is time for a conversation. Conversation, dialogue and exchange enable us to find agreement, and to find our authenticity again.

Asking for help

It is often difficult for many of us to ask for help, especially if it is not in our cultural habit to do so. But, as we have just seen, asking for cooperation with others is essential to experiencing joy in our birth and parenting.

So, just imagine that you could receive all the help you needed by simply asking. Allow yourself to create a vision of the support you would need to really thrive and shine in this stage of your life. Then, go out and ask for it!

What aspects of your birth preparation would benefit from cooperating from others? Here are some areas to consider:

- Who could provide practical help before and/or after the birth with shopping, cooking, cleaning and childcare? Make a post-birth wish list of people who will help you with a particular task on a given day.
- Who would be a good person to voice your fears and anxieties to, who would sit with you and listen to your birth story in an open and loving way?
- Who will offer you positive words of encouragement as you make your way through your choices and find a path that is right for you?

- Who could act as your birth mentor?
- Who could you go to for some nurturing? A massage, a home cooked meal lovingly prepared and served, a hug when you need it?
- Who could act as your mothering mentor? Who inspires you? Who could help you be the mother you want to be? Who will encourage you to find your own way through and to have fun along the way?
- Who could act as a fathering mentor? Who inspires you? Who could help you to be the father you want to be? Who will encourage you to find your own way through and to have fun along the way?

You might find any of these people among your loved ones, friends, relatives, colleagues or you might have to go out looking for them, either by hiring professional support or through local groups. When you start looking, you will find the person who is in the right place at the right time to help you, just take it one step at a time, starting with little asks if that's easier and moving onto bigger asks as you become more confident.

Prayer

Whatever name we choose to give it – God, Spirit, Love, Universe, the Divine, or any variation on that theme – at some stage of our journey with Please it will help us to step into a place of trust and to appeal to a higher force to give us strength on our journey. Prayer may carry all kinds of emotive connotations, but really it is just shorthand for saying Please in a sacred atmosphere. In offering up a prayer, we are attempting to align our passion and vision with the will of God. If we find some resistance to the concept of God and prayer, then it may be helpful for us to momentarily suspend our judgment – to decide neither to agree or disagree with the idea of prayer, to simply to choose to stay open and let the thought float around in our consciousness for a while.

Regular quiet time or a meditation practice may help us to rest into prayer. Creating sacred spaces in our lives can be simple: it could be that 10-minute walk through the park before we catch a bus to work, the moment we take to sit and pause before we eat our lunch in the middle of a busy day or a long soak in a warm bath before bed. Or it may be a regular yoga class or a more formal sitting meditation practice at home. All of these gestures create a space in which we are free from distraction and in which we gift ourselves with a few moments peace in which we can connect with our heart.

Finding stillness is very nourishing, yet it is an often neglected skill in modern society. It allows us to experience that sense of interconnectedness that makes the mind both strong and clear. Practising stillness relaxes the body too, and through meditation, or regularly pausing to notice our breath and to clear our mind, we are not only able to de-stress but we are also able to dip into the realms of inspiration, intuition, revelation, creativity and illumination.

Prayer is magical and prayer is passionate, and love is a vital ingredient of both magic and passion. Loving the divine within ourselves enables us to love the divine within others and thereby feel more unity in our lives. Through prayer we connect with the timelessness of humanity, while simultaneously responding to what is being asked of us as individuals here and now on this earth. Hence we are able to find solace and rest in something that is far bigger than our own ego and which provides us with the opportunity to celebrate our true life purpose. What's more, by acknowledging the baby in this process, we also affirm the baby's own special and unique purpose, and we can then trust that we are in alignment with that. This makes for a deeply connected journey for the baby, who experiences and feels so much during its time in the womb.

So, when we form a clear vision of our birth and parenting, follow that through with intention, cooperating with others along the way, and pray for the good of all then we clear a way for the baby to get in touch with their own purpose, unhampered by our personal expectations and agendas. In this way, the fifth secret of a joyful birth unlocks the potential joy of embodiment and birthing for the both baby and its parents. This brings happiness to all members of the family and lays strong foundations of love, clear and open communication and a strong connection to heart as we make our passage into parenting.

Say a little prayer
Make time every day or once a week to light a candle, an act that will help you remember clearly that you have a vision and what your intentions are as you prepare for birth and parenting. Ask for courage on this journey; ask for well-being for your baby, and for strength and grace in your birthing.

Case Study 5: *Goodbye, Sorry*

Julia

Julia came for a session when she was about 30 weeks pregnant with her first child. Her body was not comfortable and she was experiencing pelvic pain that meant she had had to give up her job as a gardener earlier than she had thought. She felt over whelmed by stuff she had to do and was worried that she wasn't "up to the job".

We did the questionnaire and the questions that drew attention were in the "moving on" bit of Goodbye and the releasing old resentments bit of Sorry. She felt all this old relationship stuff was coming up for her that was affecting how she felt in her pregnancy. This showed itself as "naggy, picky, criticisms" which made her feel bad and didn't engender good feeling in the home. She was worried about hygiene standards, which Julia realized were like the voice of her mother coming out. She was also feeling very alone and isolated. She had recently moved out of the city to a more rural area where she had moved in with her partner. This meant she wasn't so close to friends and support she was used to.

When we looked at this further Julia remembered that as a child she had moved a lot, three times to new areas and schools, all at important transitional times. So we looked at the fact that she seemed to have experienced transitions as a time of isolation and fear and pulling back into herself. This was further complicated in the way that before she had been pregnant she had felt resentment at any friends who were pregnant and complaining of difficulty. This is because she had at that time felt it was unfair of them to complain when they were so lucky to be pregnant. So now she held back from inviting her old friends into her world, feeling sensitive if they didn't have kids that she may be making them feel sad or resentful. In this way she had also slightly excluded herself from what she called "the pregnancy club" as previously she had felt resentful she hadn't belonged to this club. With her moving so many times as a child this had also had the effect of making her resistant to clubs and cliques she hadn't often felt welcomed into them. With this realization (Goodbye) she made a decision. With this realization (Goodbye) she made a decision to let that go and invite her friends into her world and be honest. Remembering the sadness she had felt at being excluded as a child, and also later as an adult when she felt excluded from the "pregnancy club", gave her a chance to let all that go and embrace where she was now with joy and excitement.

The next time I saw her she had "given in with abandon" to the pregnancy world and received support from her friends. This also had the knock on effect of her being less critical of her partner and not taking out her previous isolation on him. She was approaching the birth in a much freer and more supported way. Her daughter was born at home in water with much enjoyment and delight soon after the second session. She felt more empowered and stronger than ever before in her life. However, meeting up after the birth she stated she had taken for granted that this new-felt power and confidence would remain as she learnt to parent. It took Julia by surprise that she was hounded by doubt – "why did you think you could do this?" and "here I am being crap again" – so those old stories of feeling overwhelmed and not up to the job resurfaced. Doing the same work of letting go of old critical internal voices helped her to find out who she was when she wasn't going down the path of old insecurities. Parenting a baby after birth is another transition and given that transitions were so isolated and difficult earlier in her life, it is perhaps no surprise that self-belief at a time of probably one of the biggest transitions in life was more challenged than ever before. Being conscious of this helped, and as she opened herself to being in a new, different place, Julia witnessed the child in her growing up to parent her child. It is with the state of Goodbye we can sometimes learn something about the way we do transitions, and it is within the state of Sorry that we can heal old stories and old wounds that don't serve us any longer.

"

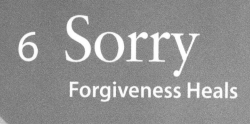

6 Sorry

Forgiveness Heals

Secret six is about refining our awareness of who we are and the stories we bring to our journey. It is about clearing the way of the future by healing the hurts of the past. Secret six is Sorry. When we meet Sorry in pregnancy, we are invited to see and act with humility, to recognise where we need to patch up our past and make amends, with ourselves and others, and no-one else can do this for us. We cannot meet Sorry, therefore, without a strong sense of personal responsibility; not blame, not guilt, but rather a knowing that, as we come into contact with other people, we alone are responsible for ourselves. We must tread lightly with our words, opinions, intentions and actions, repairing any broken bridges in our relationships where necessary.

Sorry

Life is a series of relationships. We do not exist in isolation and we could not live in complete isolation, even if our relationships are not close ones we depend on others in a myriad of ways to make our daily lives possible – the food we eat, the clothes we wear, the services we use, the books we read, the films we watch, the creation and consumption of these and almost every other aspect of our lives are huge feats of human relationship and cooperation. Each of us also has a part to play within our own unique circle of life.

Most of us are lucky enough to have immediate family, extended family, friends, colleagues and neighbours. If we never rubbed up against anyone, said or did something that provoked an uncomfortable response in another, or if we strove to please everyone all of the time, then we would lack any potential for growth in our lives. That is not to say that we should swagger around with the desire to come into conflict with others. But, we should not shy away from challenges, since every challenge is a chance to learn something about ourselves and others.

Moreover, every challenge offers us an opportunity in which we can find the best way to meet and to, where possible, resolve any discord in a peaceful way. This is Sorry. Even if we are not always successful in every situation, by acknowledging our responsibility, by showing willing to express remorse and then finding a way to repair any broken bridges, we will be able to release old habits and create more nourishing conditions for fruitful relationships. Within this context we will feel more supported and feel more able to approach birth and parenting in freedom, lightness and joy.

Pregnant Pause

In pregnancy, we are much softer and more yielding emotionally. Tears flow more freely and we have a greater urge to express how we're feeling. Without even trying, then, we have already landed in an ideal state in which to meet Sorry. This is beneficial not only to ourselves, but of course to our baby.

By having an emotional clear out, which is something we may have already begun to experience with the help of those vivid dreams that many of us get in pregnancy, then we clear the way for our birth and parenting and we clear the way for our baby. Babies come to us with the beauty of innocence. It is our responsibility, therefore, that we ensure they are not festering in old wounds and hurts which we have pushed beneath the surface and kept ourselves disconnected from.

Each wound may have its own story, a story of shame, self-criticism, guilt, fear, self-loathing or even abuse. In relation to our own family of origin there may be areas in which we still hold blame or attacking thoughts. Or, quite simply, we might still be carrying around ideas about ourselves that are no longer truthful, yet we are still living out. Indeed, there may be real reason for us to harbour such thoughts and feelings. Yet, as long as we keep reacting to them, rather than responding to them thoughtfully and kindly, pausing each time to notice how they affect us and what harm that continues to do to us, then we will not be able to approach birth with the freedom it deserves.

We may not be able to heal every hurt, or to make peace with every demon during our pregnancy – this may be part of the process of our parenting journey, which will of course present a lifetime of challenges. But pregnancy is the place to make friends with Sorry, to make friends with ourselves, to bring peace to our story. If we are at least aware of what has been going on for us, then we can bring forgiveness to ourselves as the forerunner of bringing forgiveness to others. We need to give ourselves permission to get it wrong, to realise that we have made mistakes and for that to be OK. After all, birth and parenting are not pass or fail experiences, and we have nothing to prove, least of all to ourselves. All is required is that we show up for the job and do the best we can, with the willingness and humility of one who truly dedicates themselves to their work.

Loosening Our Grip

Human beings are incredibly resilient and creative. There is no experience that we can't handle. Given the right support and being allowed to enjoy an atmosphere of loving kindness and respect (we create this for ourselves, in our own minds, regardless of whether others provide this for us or not) there is nothing that we need to hide from ourselves. Our bodies are softening thanks to the hormone relaxin, which is released in pregnancy, and our hearts are too. If we brace ourselves against the imagined pressures of birth and parenting, keep burying and locking fears and hurts away, then they may come to the surface much more loudly further along in our pregnancy, or during our birth or early parenting.

So, if we are having trouble letting go of hurt, then this may be the point at which we ask for help with doing so, professional or otherwise. It may be useful to think about how we have let go of things in the past – perhaps on reflection we realise all the things we are still holding onto! Women hold a lot of their emotions in their pelvic region, it is like a cauldron of experiences and secrets. There may be stories around menarche (first menstruation), our first sexual experiences, losing our virginity, abortion, miscarriage and sexuality, each of which may leave its mark on the body. Bringing love and acceptance to these stories, voicing them where necessary and dissolving negative self-perceptions will help us to feel more relaxed in ourselves. This, by turn, will enable us to relax our muscles and pelvis on a deeper, physical level when it comes to birthing our baby. We need to be as open as possible to birth our baby, and we need to be as open as possible to meeting each baby's individual needs in parenting. This openness and acceptance is what allows us to experience true joy in our birth and parenting.

Keywords

Who steers the course of our lives? Who do we blame when things go wrong? Do we bury our heads in the sand when we meet challenge? Do we expect to be rescued? For someone else to make everything better for us? All these are questions of responsibility, the first keyword of Sorry. When we recognise our agency, our responsibility in life, then we can start to move towards making amends, looking after our relationships, looking after and loving ourselves, which leads us through remorse, repair and, finally, release.

Responsibility

In Western culture there is a fierce connection between responsibility, blame and guilt. If we are responsible for something, then we must be to blame, we must accept our guilt, we must take the rap. It's no wonder then, that many of us approach life with a defensive attitude. After all, if we admit to doing something wrong, something which had an impact on others, then we lay ourselves open to all kinds of criticism. In doing this, we constantly nip and tuck the image of ourselves that we project to others, hiding away and cutting off parts of ourselves in case others cast blame or tell us we got something wrong. This is completely different understanding of responsibility than the one we want to foster here. Nothing about it is helpful for our growth as individuals.

It is much more helpful to think of responsibility as a coming back to self. By this we mean approaching our relationships with an awareness that allows us to notice what is happening and what our reaction is to each situation. This enables us to see what part we play in creating or undoing tension in our relationships. We learn something new about ourselves, which we acknowledge and accept with love and kindness, and we also begin to develop empathy for others as we become aware that we cannot understand everything that is going on within a particular individual at any given time. With this sense of compassion for ourselves and others, we can let go of blame and commit to being less reactionary, more responsive in the future.

If we find particular conversations or relationships difficult, we can stop and pause for a moment to perhaps try and understand what is pushing our buttons. It maybe that it touches on an old hurt or story within us. Then, it becomes less about the other person bugging us and more about where needs some love and attention within ourselves. As long as we keep ignoring that part of ourselves, though, the other person will keep pushing our buttons, aggravating us, making us angry and upset. We may need to put boundaries around our relationship if it is harmful or abusive, but it is also part of our choice to respond mindfully to the situation rather than to continue to react against it.

Saying Sorry

I was once told by a young Lithuanian woman that, as a woman approaches birth, it is the tradition in her village for the pregnant woman to go from house to house to make peace with anyone she needs to. This stems from the belief that a woman cannot free herself to birth until she has freed herself from past resentments.

When it comes to saying 'Sorry', rather than feeling burdened by guilt and shame, you can cast your apology in a different light. Instead of saying 'I'm sorry, I was wrong, I'm guilty, a bad person', you could try: 'I'm sorry that my words or actions upset you. I regret that I was insensitive and I feel sad that I caused distress.' It is always better to say sorry and make your peace than to carry around bitterness and resentment – it might not change the past but it will enrich the future.

Responsibility, therefore, goes hand in hand with being responsive. Responsibility need not be the burden it is made out to be, it is merely the ability to respond. The importance of acquiring this skill for birth and parenting cannot be underestimated. Birth asks us to really know ourselves, to know that we can go within ourselves and meet whatever we find there with love and acceptance. If we keep hiding away from ourselves, then however much we prepare intellectually and physically for birth, we run the risk of sabotaging our birth experience because we have not woken up to who we really are. We birth how we live and we live how we birth, and our attitudes, beliefs and level of self-understanding and acceptance are all integral to this.

Countless times women have told us that they thought they had done all they could to prepare for birth, but when it came to the birth they began to close up against the experience, they became fearful of feeling. They wanted to push the experience away, to numb themselves to it. They may have had the natural birth they wanted, or they may not, but what remained with them most strongly were the feelings around the experience and at some point in labour they may have been asked to go to a place within themselves that they really didn't want to face. So, while it is not always easy or achievable to tie up all the loose ends and messy feelings, it will be incredibly helpful in our birthing if we can at the very least acknowledge where our tender points are, notice the bits about ourselves and our lives that we find difficult to be with and be prepared for them to make themselves known in our birthing. If we make friends with our shadow now, during our pregnancy, then we can invite and welcome it to come along for the ride in a more conscious way. This is a most human, life-giving journey, so why not embrace and celebrate all of our humanness in our birthing?

We need to practise responsibility, to exercise our ability to respond in labour and in parenting. In labour we can notice when it is getting strong, when we are experiencing its full force and how we respond to that – do we tense up and fight or do we go with it, accept and surrender? In parenting we can notice when it gets tough, perhaps when a child's needs or neediness touches a place in us where our own needs were or are not being met, and either react with anger or choose to respond with love. If we keep hiding away from the full colour of our experience, or put too much pressure on ourselves to get it right, then we are not supporting ourselves, we are not being kind. When we know what we bring, or are in some way open to being curious about finding out more about what we bring, then we can be more discerning in our responses, in our intentions and in our actions. During this process we will discover that there are clearly some things that need to be dealt with now, and others that will be important to give attention to at a later stage when we have the resolve. Wearing our responsibility well, is like travelling with a well-thought out backpack – there's everything in there that we need to get us through most situations, and nothing in there that is not helpful, that will weigh us down and tire us out. The freer and lighter we feel, the more energy we will have to enjoy the trip.

When considering what we need to take responsibility for when approaching our birth it may be wise to remember that our earliest physiology was shaped by our earliest experience. Much research today suggests that our own birth is laid down in the cell memory of our body, and though we may not consciously "remember" it, the memory is there all the same. The usefulness of this suggestion might be that you find out something about your birth (mum and dad), and so you can understand something about what you may be bringing to this birth. You also have the chance to learn something about that first great journey that you made, all those years ago. You can then name it as your journey, not your baby's, and your baby may be freed up to make their own journey! Sometimes I hear women say "oh all the women in my family find birth painful…."Or "all the women in my family are always induced…" and I wonder at the usefulness of this kind of assumption. It can easily be a self-fulfilling prophecy, and does not allow you to make conscious choices along the way that support your own authentic way of doing it. Sometimes we have "to know" what is there before we can even attempt to let it go, or stop it from inhibiting the freedom of the present. We can become reactive rather than responsive.

Sticky Situations

One way of discovering where you may be stuck in your life, where you may not be exercising full responsibility, is to start noticing what experiences come your way. What people or situations press your buttons – it may be a surprise to learn that not everyone finds the same things as irritating as you do? What triggers fear instead of joy? What conversations do you keep mulling over long after they've finished? What people continue to rile you even when you're not in their company? Be curious, not self-critical. Notice where you're not taking responsibility, where something might be touching a place within you that causes you to react rather than to respond.

As soon as we discover that we are pregnant, then, we are clearly in a place of responsibility. It is our baby, no-one else's. Even if the father is not involved, two people made this baby and both people must meet their responsibility. The choices and decisions that we make must support the whole family. We can only do our best, nothing more, nothing less. It is our duty and obligation to act responsibly in all situations, and this may ask us to grow up at an unprecedented rate as we become parents. Now, that is the real challenge.

Remorse

Remorse is that uncomfortable feeling that we have done something that has caused upset or distress for ourselves or another. When we actively allow ourselves to feel remorse, as opposed to shrinking away from it and ignoring the situation, we take responsibility for our actions and then feel the sadness that comes from acknowledging that we have caused pain. This is not about whether we caused pain intentionally or not (doesn't matter) or whether we did anything wrong (not relevant), we are merely recognising that our actions have caused an upsetting response.

In pregnancy, we might feel remorse when we acknowledge that we continue to behave in ways within the couple relationship that are not kind or respectful. We might be so absorbed in ourselves, our changing body, our symptoms, our changing life, that we cannot fully embrace the experience of the baby inside or involve our partner in the journey. We might have had an abortion previous to this pregnancy, feel immense guilt, and have all kind of worries about whether this baby will be alright, whether we deserve to have a healthy baby after an abortion. We might discover at a scan that the baby's gender is not the one we hoped for and feel guilty that we feel this way. Or, we might be a subtle sense that our past habits and fears, or the role we have rigidly assigned to ourselves in birth, is getting in the way of our ability to approach labour and birth as free and relaxed as we would like to be.

We can experience any number of scenarios and feel remorse in all kinds of different ways, but none of this means we have done something wrong and it certainly doesn't call for harsh, or even mild, self-criticism. Indeed, the opposite is true. We need to see what is happening, take responsibility for that, feel the sadness, explain what has been going on, and extend love to everyone involved, including ourselves.

Just knowing that we can give ourselves permission to recognise our responsibility and then to feel remorse and sadness, can bring about a great sense of relief. So, we stop trying to get it right, we notice what's going on, what the pattern is, we take responsibility, feel the remorse and move onto the next stage. We need to have the courage to be honest with ourselves, to accept our weaknesses and to be willing to work with them. Life is a constant state of flux and change, that is the only thing that is guaranteed in pregnancy and parenting. We all have the potential to trip up and bring about an experience or result that we didn't want. Sometimes it's like we can't stop ourselves, either. Thankfully, though, conscience acts as a sharp cattle prod. When we feel its prick, we know there's something we need to refine about how we are in relationship, in life. This helps us to move towards freedom and joy.

This means we can start to let go of our hurts and wounds without shutting them up, hiding them away, and worrying if they'll come back to haunt us later (more about this below).

Repair

Once we've accepted responsibility and felt remorse, the next step is repair. The first two steps are important, sure, but they're pretty pointless without then seeking to repair the damage we've done. OK, so it wasn't our intention to hurt someone through our words or actions, but if we did then we need to patch things up. And, if we don't know how to do that, what do we do? We ask the person involved what we can do to make amends. Once we've said sorry and shown remorse, this is the natural follow on, however difficult it may feel at the time.

When it's our unborn baby, however, it may feel a little strange to ask them what we need to do to make amends. This is where listening to our heart or voice of intuition, and being open to the response, helps. This will help us to imagine what is needed and to put ourselves in our baby's place. We might apologise and acknowledge, for instance, that we have been preoccupied with other things, that we have been stressed and feeling disconnected from baby. We might then make a commitment to finding ways to feel more supported and so reduce our stress levels.

With a new baby that cries a lot, we may need to be open enough to allow their experience of birth to be acknowledged. We may be able to respond easily to their needs crying – I'm hungry, I've got a wet nappy, I'm tired, I need a cuddle – but we culturally we may find it less comfortable to be with a baby who is simply crying out to be heard. A lot of energy goes into shushing babies with constant rocking, the use of mechanical rocking chairs and cots, the offering of a dummy, breast or bottles, when what they might actually be expressing is a memory of their birth or an experience in the womb. Perinatal educator, Karlton Terry (see www.ippe.info), describes this as 'memory crying,' which has the purpose of releasing a particular experience. This might be the memory of the stress they felt when mum and dad were having a hard time during pregnancy, the compression of passing through the birth canal, a headache resulting from the use of forceps, the newness of being in the world outside the comforting containment of the womb. By listening to and hearing our babies in this way, we will be helping to repair the earliest of wounds and enable them to move forward into their lives more freely. Just learning to be with our children's tears in a compassionate way can have a profound effect on parenting.

If there are wounds to repair within ourselves – issues surrounding sexuality and shame, miscarriage, abortion, for instance – then we might decide that we would benefit from the help of a professional. This might be a counsellor or a body worker who will help us to get clearer about what it is we need in order to help us to feel more peace within ourselves. Even by gifting ourselves with a regular massage or reflexology treatment might be enough to help us to shift into a more loving relationship with ourselves, noticing where we are being less than kind.

When Your Baby Cries

If your baby continues to cry after you have attended to all its needs – fed and cuddled your baby, changed its nappy, made sure they have the sleep they need – then just stop and listen to what your baby is trying to tell you. It may be that they are 'memory crying', expressing the need to release an experience during their time in the womb or at birth that has had an impact on them. So, stop jiggling, rocking and shushing your baby, sit and be with its crying and ask yourself: What is the quality of the crying? What would they be saying if they could use words to express how they're feeling? Talk to them while you're doing this. They will apppreciate the sentiment in your tone of voice. Listening to your baby in this open and conscious way is an amazing gift for your baby. You will be welcoming them into the world in the most loving way by validating their experience as a new soul finding their feet in this new life. New parents probably can't listen with this depth of attention all the time, but offering your baby a time each day when the parents will enter "the kingdom of the baby" (Karlton Terry) and just really listen with an empathy that doesn't try and fix, but rather tries to understand something about the experience of this new being, with curiosity and connection. If your friend was trying to express some anger or sadness at having had a strong experience you would probably just listen to what they were telling you.

We might not be able to address every old wound, but even by allowing ourselves to be courageous and open to meeting them when and if they arise, we are already equipping ourselves with the love and compassion that will help us to be with whatever chooses to show up in our birthing. It might be that labour brings about all kinds of repair work in itself, since we might meet some feelings and memories that we didn't expect to. If we can trust ourselves to be with whatever comes forward, retain our humility, and know that we have every within ourselves to cope with that, then we will be able to really let go and accept that the journey will be whatever it will be. This means that, whatever form our birth takes, we will be able to grow from the experience and move forward into the next stage of our lives with greater strength and joy.

Discovering Where It Hurts

It is easy to say that we know ourselves well, that life is just fine thank you very much, to shrug off our fears and anxieties and present an image to the world that we are grounded and confident. Yet, however we live our lives, whatever our upbringing and life experiences, there is always room for us to be more aware of what we carry with us, most of which is probably quite unconscious most of the time.

Give yourself some space, some quiet time, free from distractions to consider the following questions about what you bring to your birthing. Avoid self-censorship and self-editing, just let your responses flow freely and honestly, and be curious, rather than critical, about what comes forward. Notice when you answer a question in such a way that you are trying to prove something about yourself, to yourself, be that positive or negative.

- What are you greatest fears about birth?
- What are your biggest hopes?
- What experience do you want to avoid at all costs in your birthing?
- How might that scenario link to a past experience?
- What do you most wish for in your birthing? Again, how does that link to your past?
- What pressures do you put on yourself and why? Generally, in the way you live your life? And, specifically, in relation to your birth?
- Do you allow yourself to make mistakes, to 'get it wrong'? Does this feel safe for you? If not, why not? What would happen if you slipped up?
- How do you feel about being a woman?
- What have you learnt about and from the womanly experiences of fertility, bleeding and birthing? Where have these stories come from?
- Think of a woman you admire for the way she expresses her womanhood and femininity. What qualities do you appreciate most in this woman?

- Which areas in your life do you experience guilt and self-judgment?
- In what ways do you find it hard to take responsibility?
- What do you need to do to attend to these aspects of yourself, to repair these negative self-perceptions?
- Do you need to say sorry to your baby for anything?
- Is there any way in which it has been difficult for you to be the mother you wanted to be, including during your pregnancy?
- What, if anything, gets in the way of you communing and communicating with your baby?
- Do you need to say sorry to your partner? If so, what for?
- Is there any aspect of your relationship in which you have found it difficult to take responsibility?
- What do you need to do to repair your relationship in order for both of you to experience more harmony?

Release

Sorry, like Goodbye (chapter four), is about letting go. The release that comes from acknowledging responsibility, feeling remorse, finding repair and then letting go of past hurts and self-judgments brings more grace to our lives. Through atonement and reconciliation we feel more at peace in the world, we become more forgiving of ourselves and, by consequence, more forgiving of others. This brings us back to that spiritual sense of connection to a bigger whole – when we accept ourselves and our misperceptions, then we more easily accept others. If we can accept that we may have sticky points and contradictory feelings, then we can accept these in another. If we can accept that we are human and part of our human journey is about learning what it is to be human, then we can accept others are also on a journey of their own. When we can sit with our pain and our wounds, and bring love to them, then we can sit with the wounds and pain of another and bring balm to their sores too.

Ultimately, such qualities as forgiveness and self-acceptance, allow us to rest and soften into our being. We bring a sense of wonder to all we experience and let our judgments fall away. We do not become preoccupied with how much birth preparation we are doing in comparison to others, whether our birth was a success or failure, whether our baby gets into a routine or sleeps through the night, or whether our parenting choices or methods are better than those of another. Instead, we recognise that we are just a small but unique and sparkling part of a magnificent whole. We attend only to the part that we have to play in this life, worry less about what others are doing, and live in a state of absolute responsibility for ourselves, and for our babies and children.

This realisation may bring a feeling of lightness, it may feel like a huge weight has dropped away, a burden has fallen from our previously stooped shoulders. With a more relaxed mind and body, we can then let go of control, let go of agendas, and simply be open to experience and learning. Release helps us to feel more spacious within ourselves and, happily, that brings far greater simplicity and clarity to our lives. We can be open to the 'I don't know' feeling and trust that we will find a way through. With this knowledge, acting with kindness yet knowing that our words carry an energy that can impact another however well-meaning we are, we can begin to take ourselves a little less seriously, without being flippant. After all, we are a work in progress, just like our children, so we may as well enjoy ourselves along the way. And, if we're having fun, while staying conscious and mindful of our intentions and actions, there's no doubt we'll begin to experience the great potential for joy in our birth and parenting.

Meditation On Self-Forgiveness

Find a comfortable place to sit, using cushions and wall support if you need. Take a moment to check through your body, noticing what is there, what it feels like. Bring your attention to your breath, allowing the in-breath to come into the body without grabbing at it, and letting go of tension and holding as you breathe out. Have an intention that you are going to use this time to let go of a place within you that holds some guilt or criticism about something. It could be a present day experience, or it could be something that happened a long time ago but still makes you feel a bit bad about yourself when you remember it. Try and let something just bubble up rather than forcing. Hold a strong intention that you are willing to let go of self-criticism around something that may otherwise feel heavy for you right now, and in your birthing. If you can't let it go, then at least you can ask to see it differently. So let some story or experience come forward and notice how you feel about it. In what way do you think you give yourself a hard time about it? If you were a friend telling you the same story would you similarly judge them? Can you feel yourself release the guilt, one breath at a time? Can you forgive yourself for getting it wrong (from your perception, as very possibly you didn't get anything wrong), for being less than perfect? What might you learn from this that would help you to move forward? Can you bring in a feeling of relaxation in your body as you begin to accept yourself and all that happened? What would help you to accept this experience? This may not be easy and as I said before, sometimes just being willing and open to forgiving oneself and so releasing guilt, is all we have. We don't know how to go forward with that. But bringing the idea forward is a start. You may want to visualise yourself taking the heavy experience or guilt out of your back pack and placing it down somewhere (a forest, the sea, a mountain) and then breathing into yourself and noticing lightness in your body. Visualising isn't for everyone though so don't worry if that doesn't work for you. Maybe just feeling that with every out breath you are letting that heaviness out of your body, one piece at a time. Let your body rest back, be held by the earth underneath you, and come into a place of wholeness.

This exercise can be repeated (and it often serves us to repeat it!) by mum and/or dad whenever they feel heavy or self-critical, are holding guilt or pressurizing themselves in an unhelpful way. Often we can notice this by paying attention to the body as this state of unease often feels like an uncomfortableness in your own skin.

Case Study 6: *Goodbye*

Fern

It is probably no surprise that the state of Goodbye comes up often times in working with Seven secrets of birth since giving birth is such a "goodbye" moment. Fern was a second time mum who had a three year-old daughter. We were drawn to looking at the fourth Secret of Goodbye and breaking that down to see which bit of that state presented some challenge. Fern made decisions easily. However the next bit "completion" was harder as doubt often crept in at this point. We looked at her first birth and particularly transition, which had indeed been hard. Fern realized that when she doubted herself in this way she lost connection to her "warrior woman" self that would so help these times of change. We looked at ways she could learn to trust more and not loose connection to this empowered part of herself. Indeed when she examined her decision-making to date (partner, house, education choices for her child and so on) she could see that her decision making was very good, and that she would stand by her decisions. This gave her confidence to be in the courage and inner knowing of her warrior self as she approached her birth. She made a decision to keep those people who she felt fed her doubt, away as she approached birth. She would surround herself with the people in her life who fed the confidence she now began to connect to within herself more easily. In real terms this meant asking her mum to be around to help more, and giving herself permission to not be around her mother-in-law at this time who was afraid of the idea of home birth.

As she was more conscious of making decisions and transitions and completing on them, she had the opportunity to drop underneath the "stuff" that had previously got in the way of the flow. This made the Goodbye state more flowing as she trusted herself more. Fern said it literally felt enlightening. This was then reflected in her home birth which followed. She was able to meet the challenge of labour in a way that she worked very instinctively from a confident inner place. When she needed to remind herself of that inner warrior woman she did, and remembered how it helped her find courage to meet the needs of the transition without doubt. There were times when doubt did appear in her labour but knowing that it may be familiar for her to dwell there or get stuck there for a while enabled her to again drop underneath and follow her own flow, her own decisions.

"

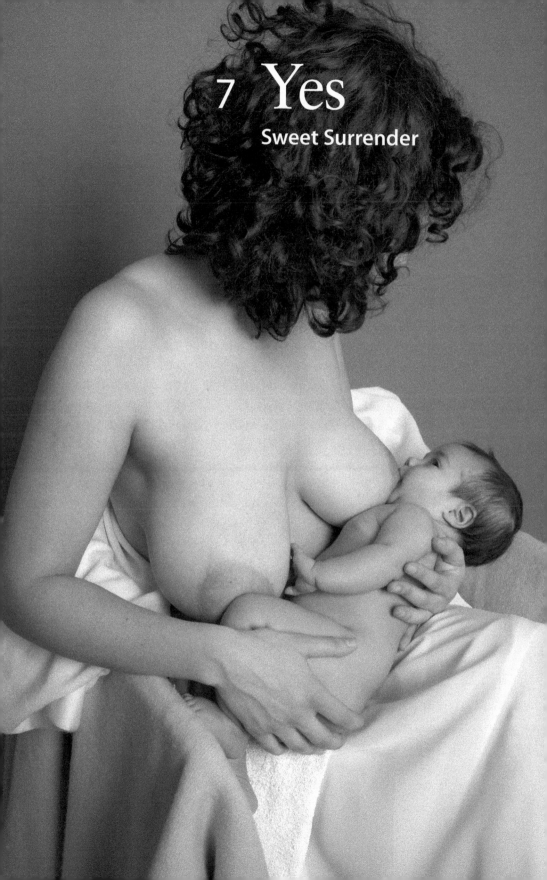

7 Yes

Sweet Surrender

The seventh and final secret of a joyful birth is Yes. By meeting Yes in our birthing, we are able to relax and find peace within ourselves as we accept the flow of life and trust where it is taking us. Approaching birth with a strong Yes, therefore, brings with it a sense of spaciousness and allowing, which is beneficial for our nervous system and supports our birthing body. It is also good for our mind, as we let go of resistances and surrender to the joy of our journey as it unfolds.

Yes

A strong No (chapter one) is the foundation of a strong Yes. When we are true to ourselves, and can be clear about what we don't want and what we do want without stepping into old habits and patterns, then we will experience a much greater degree of freedom in our life. This is a very helpful place to be in for birth – we have emptied our bag of the heavy weight of must and musn'ts, fears and agendas, and filled it with the lightness of clarity, openness and trust instead. With these qualities nourishing and supporting us, we can feel more excited about what lies ahead and enter our birth with grace and a sense of wonder and divinity. Every birth is divine, for every birth is a miracle and bringing a child into the world is an event that will move us beyond words. Nothing can prepare us for the power of this experience, so we can only wait in anticipation and fully embrace it when the moment comes.

Relax, Enjoy The Journey

Trust is implicit in Yes. Nowhere is this more apparent than in the final state of Yes, Surrender, which challenges us to completely trust in the process and be willing to go with the flow. Even if this is not our first baby, there is so much about the experience of birth that is unknown. Every birth is unique, and every woman's experience is unique. No-one can tells us what our birth will be like, however well-prepared we feel we are.

So, how can we find a place within ourselves that is willing to accept this unknown and to be OK with it? In order to do so, we have to let go of control and to let go of our desire for our birth to take a specific form. Women often say they had an 'active birth' or a 'hypno birth' or a 'natural birth', but we cannot label our birth experience except to call it our own. There is no one solution, no one right way to birth and no one way to feel about our birth. When we are in a state of Yes, we have nothing to prove and we commit to the experience with joy and surrender. This surrender is similar to falling in love, in which we allow anything to happen, we acknowledge the risks but yet the only natural thing to do is to commit to it anyway, and enjoy ourselves along the way.

Giving The Go Ahead

Imagine what it would feel like if we gave ourselves permission to approach our birth and parenting with surrender. Imagine what it would be like if we could allow ourselves to find acceptance in our journey whatever happens along the way. Imagine how much freer and relaxed we would be if we took away the pressure of having to birth or parent in a certain way. It is amazing how much energy is taken up by fear and the need to control everything that happens in our life. And it is amazing how much more energy we have when we let go of the fear and control and go with the flow in an active, engaged way.

Yet, for our Yes to be truly liberating, we need a strong No. Yes is not about not being able to say No. If we are not truthful about what we don't want, then it will be hard for us to be truthful about what we do want. When both our No and Yes are strong then we can be true to ourselves, our choices become clearer and decision-making is more straightforward.

Being Where We Are

As soon as we discover we are pregnant, we are faced with a Yes/No decision – do we want to continue the pregnancy or not? However, even if we say yes, there may be a difference in the degree to which we feel that yes – do we feel 50 per cent yes, 70 per cent or 100 per cent? This means that we can feel more or less in a place of Yes in any given moment, which may be a useful idea for us to get used to. If we can be honest about where we are, then we will be able to trust ourselves more and feel more relaxed and joyful in the process.

It may also be helpful for us to have a sense of where we are in the bigger picture. Our birth is individual to us, but birth itself is a much bigger process. We might draw solace and find more trust in the knowledge that women have birthed and parented for eons before us, after all the survival of the human race depends on it. We may feel more allowing and accepting if we sense that it may have a spiritual element or purpose about it, and that we can choose, should we wish, to be curious and open to that potential. Or, we may simply find more surrender if we trust that we are part of nature and that nature is intricately and perfectly designed for birth and new life, just like us.

Anything that enables us to feel more relaxed and which supports our ability to say Yes, therefore, is incredibly valuable. This may bring up questions about where and with whom we feel safest. During pregnancy, it is important to take time to reflect and notice where in our life we feel most supported, and where we do not. When exploring our birth choices, we need to ask ourselves with which people and in what classes do we feel most relaxed? Most joyful? Whatever it is that gives us the strength to say Yes and mean it, embrace it, and surrender to it, is a gift for our birth and parenting, a gift for ourselves and our baby.

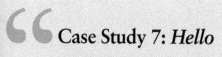

Case Study 7: *Hello*

Rebecca

Sometimes we can't fix a tricky situation but we can help bring some choice to it. Rebecca came to see me when she was 33 weeks pregnant. Her partner and the father of the baby were not in the UK as they were waiting for immigration papers to be sorted. This was causing an enormous amount of distress for both of them. When Rebecca scored herself the only question that she gave herself a very low score on was "are you giving your birth the attention it deserves". This was clearly making her miserable as she felt she wasn't able to prepare as she was so busy sorting out immigration stuff for her partner. This was made worse by the fact they were not physically able to see each other. We looked at ways of giving the birth more attention; taking time each day to just imagine the birth, and connecting to her baby in preparing for birth. She also agreed a time each day when her partner would connect to her and the baby in a simple meditation, sending love and good feelings their way as they prepared for the big event. They didn't know whether he would be able to join them in time for the birth or not and this had made the preparation difficult. I encouraged her to prepare for all eventualities and she got 2 friends as back up doulas and made sure they knew what she hoped for in labour, how she liked to be massaged and so on. Once she put all this in place she started to relax and enjoy the pregnancy more. In actual fact her partner arrived a week or so before she gave birth and they were able to work together through the labour. Highlighting the tricky situation had highlighted a need for giving more attention and communication to mum, dad and baby, and that in itself had made things feel easier. Sometimes we cannot literally change the way things are but we can find a way to work with it that better meets the needs of the moment. She came initially very upset and forlorn at being so taken up with immigration papers that she couldn't fathom giving attention to the baby or the birth. Once she had stopped enough to see how much upset this was causing her, we were able to work out a way to include baby and birth in her preparation now. This even included dad who was so far away.

Special Place

Inside each of us there is a special place in which we can connect with an inner wisdom, a wisdom that guides us and reassures us with its presence and belief in our ability to handle everything that life throws at us, gracefully and with ease. Yet, in the busy flurry of our modern lives, it can be all too easy to lose this connection with our higher Self. Pregnancy is the perfect time to re-establish this connection and to learn to trust our instinct and intuition. In order to do so it can be useful to make a special place in the outside world that reminds us of the beauty of this inner place, which we can access and rest in whenever we need to. By creating this special place for ourselves in pregnancy, we can then bring it into our labour to give us strength and to help us surrender to the process.

In pregnancy, choose something special that will remind you of everything that is amazing about you, your body and your baby in this moment. It might be a necklace you can hold, or a cushion that you sit on. Let this symbol remind you to bring presence to yourself, your baby and the sacredness of your birthing. Practice blessing your journey however it unfolds, knowing it will be special because you are special and your baby is special too.

As you approach your birthing think about how you can bring this special place into labour. You could bring the special object with you into the birthing room. You could also bring in flowers, candles (though not in hospital), use aromatherapy (frankincense, neroli, clary sage, jasmine, lavender), bring an image from the natural world that speaks to you about the awesomeness of nature, an image or object that reminds you of your connection to your baby, or something from your Blessingway ceremony (see below) that helps you feel the strength and support of your family and friends.

Beyond these ways of bringing the divine into the birthing room, reminding you of your connection to your inner Self, that place of enduring strength, serenity and wisdom, you could talk to your birth attendants about how helpful it will be for you for birth to be recognised as sacred. You can especially involve your partner in this. Indeed, give him the job of helping to create this sacred space by holding the baby in his awareness as a sentient being with its own feelings and experiences during labour, and by being an advocate for the baby. He can also play the very important role of representing and being the presence of love at the birth. I often remind fathers that theirs is the job of being Mr Love at birth, with all that entails. He can remind you how beautiful and wonderful and completely divine you are. When fathers bring such presence to birth, they too create a special place in which the miraculous can happen. The atmosphere in the room will be raised to one of love, acceptance and surrender, enabling you to connect with your inner power and to go gracefully and magically with the flow. Every father has this special job which can make the journey for his baby an easier one, as he will also be helping the mother to feel safe and be able to let go.

Keywords

Yes is one of the most relaxed states of being. It is rare to meet someone who is adept at living within the state of Yes. When we meet them, they may have luminosity about them and their company may be energising and life giving. Such a person lets go of the past easily and moves on with a fluidity that enables them to be completely present to each moment. For such people, No is as easy a place to inhabit as Yes, and we have much to learn from them.

But what can we learn about ourselves that will help us to be better at saying Yes? By working with the four keywords of Yes we can discover what the different aspects of Yes might feel like. By exploring permission, acceptance, agreement and surrender we can begin to understand where we might be in relation to our birth and parenting and how and where we might be able to build more trust into our life.

Permission

Permission is about the art of negotiation. It is about allowing something to happen, even though we may not totally agree with it – think of it as a 51 per cent Yes! Wherever there are two opposing opinions, there will be three different scenarios or outcomes available to us: dominance and submission; conflict and aggression; or, negotiation and compromise. Negotiation has to be the only way through. In birth for instance, we might find ourselves in a situation in which we can see that it is necessary to use a particular procedure which we had really wanted to avoid. We might feel very strongly that we don't want forceps or a caesarean, say, but our midwife or obstetrician feels very strongly that it is needed. One person has to give permission in order for the birth to move forward. So, we need to listen to the other person, and listen to ourselves, finding a place in which we can negotiate and finally give permission when we can trust that it is the right decision.

Negotiation may be needed at more than one point in our birthing – Do we want to be induced if we go overdue? Do we want an internal examination during labour? Do we want to use medical pain relief if the pain becomes too much? The most important thing is not whether we make the right or wrong decision (there is no right or wrong if we come from a place of love), but that we have a choice. When our choices are clear and apparent to us, then we can reflect on those choices and take an active role in decision-making. This is completely different to handing over control to others, to being a patient, to having things happen to us rather than us making things happen for us. Negotiation keeps battles out of the birthing room and enables us to find a way through.

Let's consider the following scenario as another example of working with permission, of making space for allowing in birth. A woman has planned a natural water birth at home but she discovers she has placenta praevia (her placenta is lying over her cervix making labour very risky), so a caesarean birth becomes necessary. At this point, she needs to find a place for Yes within herself or she may feel very resentful about her birth. For some women this would be deeply disappointing. But, in order to come through this experience she has to step away from her original idea of her how her birth should be and consider the needs of her baby and the views of her carers. She listens to the information she is given and makes new choices based on new information. During the process, she takes time to listen to herself and to acknowledge her baby, and to remember what things she held as most important for her in her birthing – relaxation, communication with her baby, a peaceful atmosphere – and to bring those to her elective caesarean. She has been asked to say Yes to something she really didn't want, but in doing so it is more OK than she imagined it could ever be. All of this requires negotiation and compromise about the outward form of her birth, but allows her to maintain her integrity and stay true to herself throughout.

Acceptance

We are creatures of habit. It's not often that we like being shown a path that's different to the one we had defined for ourselves. However, by bringing acceptance into our life it opens us to other possibilities, from which we can learn and grow. Sometimes it may not always have been clear that we needed to change something about ourselves. We may have become so settled into a way of being that we limit ourselves by staying firmly within our comfort zone. Often, though, we need to feel the stretch of stepping outside our comfort zone so that our world and our life can become as big and expansive as they deserve to be.

So, how can we connect with a level of trust that allows us to actively shape our life but is also flexible enough for us to accept and relax into the unknown? There is beauty in this way of being. When we have a clear vision for our life (see chapter five), for our birth, for our parenting, it will be easier to find a way forward. When we add acceptance into the equation, then we will more easily and gracefully negotiate the different possibilities that present themselves along the way. As always, humility is very helpful in this process. Humility helps us to break down and let go of our prejudices and self-judgments so that we can be more accepting of ourselves and others in this journey.

We need to give ourselves space and time to find acceptance though. Taking time out from the busy-ness of our daily life is vital if we are to learn to listen to and connect with our instinct. Stillness allows room for reflection, in which we can ask ourselves if we are holding our opinions or ideas too tightly, or if we are right to be cautious, if we can accept something from someone else (ideas, opinions, a call for action) or if we can't. If we can be with ourselves in a very honest way, then we may discover that our prejudices have been ruling our decisions and that maybe we can soften a little and relax into different takes on life. In this way, we expand our sense of Self as we begin to accept those things that once we could not tolerate. Learning to accept difference is probably one of the things that Westerners find hardest to do, and is one of the reasons we find relationships so challenging – relationships ask us to find our Yes again and again. But, finding acceptance brings peace, and peace is an amazing grounding for our birthing, for our parenting, and for our life.

When we find a peace that comes from staying actively engaged in our life but which also includes acceptance, then we will feel more grounded and nourished as a parent. Difference, like change, is one of the only constants of parenting! Our children, believe it or not, are completely different to us. They have different likes and dislikes, different tastes in film, music, food and more. Our parenting is going to be so much easier if we can develop an ability to find heartfelt acceptance in difference.

Pregnancy can highlight ways in which we need to find more acceptance in our life. For instance, a woman who is used to being very fit and active pre-pregnancy, might suddenly find that her body is telling her to slow down and find more stillness. This may contrast greatly to the image she had of herself in pregnancy, remaining fit and full of energy until full term. If she can find acceptance in the need for her body and her baby to find more stillness, then symptoms may lessen and she may feel more peaceful in herself. Pregnancy usually asks us, in one way or another, to develop a lesser known or accepted part of our self. We can resist this or find a way to work with it, and even enjoy it.

Agreement

When our Yes moves beyond acceptance to agreement, we have found harmonious alignment. It is cause for celebration – we both want the same thing! Think of agreement as that point in an affair when two people are head over heels in love and wanting, and finding it easy, to find harmony at every stage. There is a flow to this kind of love that makes it feel easy and the feeling of harmony we experience inside is reflected in our actions on the outside.

Agreement could also be seen as two people working together towards a shared goal, each clear about their own role. In birth, mother, father and baby could all be reminded of their shared goal of coming together face-to-face. Mum and dad could commit to supporting baby in any way they can along the way, bringing as much relaxation and grace as possible to the birthing room and letting baby know they are aware and conscious that baby is making a heroic journey alongside its mother. This is a commitment to saying: 'Yes, we are all here and present in this together. Yes, we welcome you, baby. Yes, we are ready for you. Yes, we will do whatever we can to make this journey as graceful as possible for you.'

Agreement has nothing to do with coercion. Agreement must be voluntary. The decision to agree must be an informed one. Informed choice is a term that we hear frequently in birth – the parents research the pros and cons of a particular option, and then decide what would work best for them as individuals and as a couple. When we make an informed choice based on cooperation and agreement then we can feel greater intimacy with and respect for our partner. Indeed, when we find easy agreement with our partner, an agreement that has no sense of compromise and every sense of Yes, then we may be well on our way to surrender. We can begin to let go of our ego attachments and instead commit ourselves to a greater goal, the birth of our baby, and the birth of a new sense of ourselves.

Blessingway Ceremony

The Blessingway ceremony originates from the Navajos of North America. A 'baby shower' is today's version of the Blessingway. Rather than showering the baby with material gifts, though, the Blessingway blessed the baby's way into the world, celebrating the mother, baby and father in their birthing and giving them the gift of support from their extended family and friends. It also helped to connect everyone with a sense of divine wonder and the miraculousness of birthing new life, and encouraged a sense of spiritual surrender in the woman.

Traditionally, all the women who had birthed before them – sisters, mothers, grandmothers, aunts, friends – would gather together with the pregnant woman so that she could lean into their comfort and support. Women would change their hair style for the ceremony, symbolising that they were about to embark on a journey that would transform and change them forever. Only the women would attend the ceremony itself. They would then join with the men for the feasting and party. The men sometimes had their own rituals with their male family and friends to prepare them for their passage into parenthood too.

Today, a Blessingway is an opportunity for you to create ceremony and ritual about your birth and rite of passage into motherhood in a way that suits your needs and is meaningful for you. This might involve gathering together with your female friends to share stories and inspirations around birth. You could have your feet washed in a bath of relaxing herbs and oils by your midwife or doula – wild lettuce and lavender make a lovely pre-birth footbath when approaching your due date. Or you may ask your friends to each give you a bead that you can put on a string and hold at those times during your labour that you want to remember the strength offered by your circle of women friends. At the ceremony, you might feast, sing, meditate, pray, give gifts of cards and poems, with words of support and encouragement that will help you along the way. You might like to ask your friends to each commit to a job such as cooking a meal after the baby is born or to come and do some cleaning and chores around the house once or twice during the first six weeks, or beyond. Whatever you do, it is important to remember the original intention of the Blessingway, which is to connect you to the cycles of life and to help give you strength in this huge transition in your life. So, with this in mind, you could make the ceremony as simple as lighting a candle with your partner or as big as a party with lots of family and friends. However, big or small your Blessingway such ritual and symbolic gesture is a beautiful way to mark this change, to make a commitment to your journey ahead and to honour your new family.

Surrender

Softening into a place of surrender is the ideal state for our body and mind to be in as we approach birth and parenting. There is no doubt it will make our journey easier. By letting go of rigid attachments to what our birth should be like, we can use our new found energy to focus on each moment and be ready to respond to what is asked of us from a place of freedom and spiritual connection.

With surrender, we give up our own sense of self-importance and begin to realise the reality of our unity with this new life, our baby, and all of life. We let go of resistance and drop into a place within ourselves that knows that all we have to do is go with whatever shows itself, making sure that we get the rest and support we need to stay connected to the sacredness of what is unfolding. We needn't be religious to feel connected to the sacredness of birth – as we touched on before, it may simply be that you feel a connection to all the women who have birthed before you and who are birthing with you, or a connection to nature, or a deep connection to your baby. In this place we trust the bodymind to do what it needs to, without trying to control or manipulate. We trust our femininity, our body guided by our heart, and let go of any desire to overthink or analyse.

Letting go of our thinking brain, the neo-cortex part of our brain, is entirely supportive for our birthing. The hormones of labour and birth (oxytocin and endorphins) are released by the primitive, animal brain, the part of our brain that is connected to instinct and feeling. This process is inhibited by engaging with the thinking, analysing neo-cortex brain. The hormones of labour are also the hormones of love, so birth is a kind of falling in love, a form of sweet surrender.

So, if we can go with the flow then we can find even more trust in the knowledge that our body will respond positively releasing an intoxicating cocktail of helpful hormones. We can then react less and less to our labour, and choose more and more to let go, soften and melt the resistance of our bodymind. If we need something to help us with this, then it can be as simple as reminding ourselves to let go with the outbreath. Letting go with the outbreath will help release tension and resistance one breath at a time, each time returning to surrender, to relaxation and to a state of Yes.

Letting Go With The Outbreath

Our breath is one of our greatest allies in labour. It is the most efficient way of practising surrender, of allowing ourselves to go with the flow. As we let go with the outbreath, we release our diaphragm and our pelvic floor. This helps the cervix to dilate with ease. Whenever we let go with the outbreath, we let go of resistance in our mind and our body. In will be of great benefit to us if we can practise letting go with the outbreath in pregnancy. Here's how.

Sit quietly for ten minutes every day. Focus you attention solely on the outbreath, let the inbreath take care of itself, receiving it in a relaxed way. As you let go of the outbreath, imagine yourself letting go of any tension you are holding in your mind and body. You may simply visualise this release, or you may actually feel the tension dissolving. Allow this process to happen incrementally.

As you let go and release tension with your outbreath, scan your body starting with those parts closest to the ground – your pelvis, your legs. Begin by feeling like you are loosening the muscles and ligaments from the joints, releasing through your hips and groins, and widening through the pelvis. You may feel like your sacrum, the triangular bone at the base of your spine, wants to have a nice long sigh.

Let the outbreath be as free and unhampered as possible. Don't force it to be longer than you think it should be. Just stay with the possibility that your outbreath will teach you the art of surrender. Now, imagine that as you breath out, a warm knowing hand is smoothing down the back of the pelvis and either side of your spine, reminding you to let go. Continue by bringing awareness to other parts of your body, loosening, widening and smoothing, feeling for release and happy sighs.

This kind of letting go is active relaxation, it is not a collapse, but rather something that invites you to be more alive and to find strength inside yourself, from your core. Be gentle with yourself, the busy mind and body may need plenty of kind encouragement and reminders to keep letting go, and to keep letting go. Through this surrender and letting go with the outbreath, you can nurture the possibility of connecting with yourself in a different way.

As well as the thinking brain, our survival instinct can also get in the way of surrender. This is important to know. While adrenalin, the fight or flight hormone, is needed in the second stage of labour when we push our baby out, it is not useful for us in the first stage of labour. Just as the presence of adrenalin can inhibit the arousal stages of making love, it can also inhibit the dilating of the cervix during the first stage of labour. Adrenalin goes hand in hand with fear and resistance, and it can make us feel dense rather than lighter at a time when we are melting our body to let our baby through. In labour we need to be able to feel a sense of expansion, not contraction and, even if we do not believe it is possible, to be willing and to trust that we can go with whatever is asked of us. Letting go with our outbreath is one way of showing this willing. Breath by breath, moment by moment, we surrender a little more than we realised was possible. We don't have to surrender everything in one go, but we do need courage to surrender even in the face of such fears as 'If I keep letting go will it eventually overwhelm me? Will it be more than I can cope with?'

Yet fear is a simple speculation of the mind and, in birth, the mind doesn't always know what to do. It is challenged to let go and our thinking brain does not always find this comfortable. But if we continue to hold tight and not to choose the path of surrender, then our muscles and our whole body will tighten around that thought. This may make our contractions more painful, which may then feed into more fear. If we loosen our mind, however, then we will loosen our cervix. Sound can be an ally for us here.

Making deep low sounds with the outbreath help to relax the cervix and help us to stay more inside ourselves. Indeed, many spiritual traditions use sound or mantra to help people to move away from their everyday life into a more sacred place within. Sound bypasses the thinking brain and takes us to the place we need to be more quickly and far more easily than all the information and thinking in the world could do. Sound, with the breath, guides us inside ourselves, taking us by the hand and leading us onwards in our birthing.

The mantra or sound we make doesn't have to be anything special, just a surrender to the sound that wants to come through us. Let those sounds be long and low and they will vibrate through our whole body, encouraging our tissues to let go. We can let those sounds transport us to a scared place, a place where we can be in wonder of the glory of being alive and the glory of bringing life into the world. Let sound bring joy into our birthing, or if no sounds come, let the word 'surrender' simply be our mantra, reminding us of all that we have chosen in this great and joyful journey towards meeting our baby.

Roaring Like A Lion

In labour the intensity of contractions can be quite a distraction from the outbreath, from the commitment to letting go. Having support from someone who understands the need for a pregnant woman to relax and to surrender to her body is therefore a big help. This person needs to be someone the pregnant woman can trust and whose love and kindness are palpable. In order for a woman to find surrender in her birthing, she might need to bray like a donkey, roar like a lion, moan like a woman in the throes of making love, and all the sounds in between.

If you are able to express what you are feeling in labour through sound in a way that helps you to relax, not tighten, then the intensity of the contractions will diminish almost as soon as they are felt. This can be like riding a storm, with lulls and smooth waters at times, but with the ferociousness and wildness of a ten force gale at others. But surrender is surrender and the breath and sound can take you there. You don't have to control, you just have to go. Let your body be your guide, it is supremely wise.

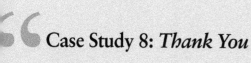

Case Study 8: *Thank You*

Helen

Helen came to see me when 28 weeks pregnant. She was fed up and depressed, as she was feeling physically uncomfortable and not enjoying her pregnancy. This meant she inhabited a constant state of discontent which didn't feel very joyful and was putting stresses on her relationship. She felt her partner wasn't doing enough to support her and that also made her feel resentful. Perhaps no surprise then that in the questionnaire the third Secret of Thank You came up. She acknowledged that she didn't appreciate her pregnancy but resented the way it made her feel.

We looked at some of the underlying reasons her body was showing certain symptoms so she could understand it from a physiological perspective and how the hormones that may be causing her discomfort were also sustaining her pregnancy and getting her pelvis ready for birth. Not appreciating her pregnancy made it hard to value it by giving it some time and attention. We looked at when she did feel better in herself and how she might up the time and energy around supporting her pregnant self.

Helen left the first session intending to start with just that. When she came back she was feeling a lot more positive and because the resentment was less she was also able to put her partner and baby into the appreciative loop. This made a sort of feedback loop as her partner then felt able to step in and support her more whereas before he had felt shut out and criticized. Good feeling grew and though Helen still had to be mindful of supporting her pregnancy symptoms she also felt able to relax more into it and receive the support that was there for her in a way she hadn't before in her life.

Helpful Resources

www.relaxedbirthandparenting.com
Find local classes, doulas, antenatal yoga, birth preparation workshops, Seven Secrets of birth and parenting workshops, professional training, and free e-newsletter and events. Birth Relaxation CD and *Seven Secrets of a Joyful Birth* book also available through this website. To contact Dominique for Seven Secrets Professional Birth Training, workshops, couple counselling and craniosacral sessions contact 07969 204 763 or email dominique@relaxedbirthand parenting.com.

www.activebirth.com
Active Birth Founder Janet Balaskas. Local classes/listing, workshops, professional training, water birth info and more.

www.borndirect.com
Internet shop, books on natural parenting, slings, nappies, bras and huge array of quality products for babies and parents.

www.7words.co.uk
7 words system created by James Burgess.

www.fatherstobe.org
Birth education for fathers.

www.craniosacral.co.uk
The Craniosacral Therapy Association, has listings of practitioners, who may help with pregnancy wellbeing and also treat babies after birth (so helping with symptoms of discomfort and breastfeeding issues).

www.ippe.info
Institute for Pre and Prenatal Education, Karlton Terry.

www.leticiavalverdes.com
Photographer who is also a doula.
Contact her at leticia.valverdes@gmail.com

www.karnikeogh.com
Contact the *Seven Secrets of a Joyful Birth* photographer at
karnikeogh@hotmail.com.

www.birthchoice.com
Info for women and fathers in where to have their baby.

www.primalhealthresearch.com
Research institute into the prenatal and baby stages of life.

www.homebirth.org.uk
Lots of research-based info on homebirth.

www.aims.org.uk
Association for Improvement in the Maternity Services, lots of good
info around birth.

www.birthasweknowit.com/10_minute_promo.html
Inspirational birth video free to watch.

www.independentmidwives.org.uk
Independent midwives in the UK.

www.moontime.co.uk
Natural products for mum and baby.

www.welcomeworldcafe.com
Healer and herbalist Amanda Rayment, pregnancy and postnatal
specialist and supplier of herbs and teas.

Acknowledgements

As in any birth there is a community that surrounds the labouring woman and helps her through. I have certainly had this in birthing this book! My three children Ezra, Arlo and Elma taught me much about birth from the inside, and for that I am eternally grateful to each one of them. My husband Mark who knows and accepts what it is to be married to a woman who is passionate about birth. My co-founder of Relaxed Birth and Parenting who inspires and supports me, thank you champion of women Louise Bennett. James Burgess who created the 7 Words system with his very brilliant and clear mind, and then generously with our colleague Richard Grey helped make sure the book used the 7 Words system in a way that was true. Jessica Adams who did a brilliant job of editing the book, making sense of my writing and trimming it into something that was more user-friendly whilst also respecting my voice, as well as giving me deadlines that meant the book got written. Janet Balaskas who trained me over twenty years ago and gifted me with a knowing of quite how far are the reaches of birth on a woman and her family. My parents for birthing me and my extended family (coming from an Anglo-Irish family there are many) who always offer enthusiasm and a sense of the possible. My colleagues Matthew Appleton and Jenni Meyer and Amanda Rayment for teaching me much about birth as well as myself. Thank you to Sue Learner independent midwife who attended my last birth all those years ago and continues to inspire, challenge and guide midwives and health professionals, doulas and pregnant women. All the women and men who offered themselves as case studies (many more than there is room for in this book and I learnt from all of you), and all the families who offered themselves for photoshoots. My photographer Karni Keogh who gave what I intended with so much grace and beauty. Karlton Terry for all he teaches me about babies, and how generously he shares what he knows. Helen Hart at SilverWood Books who has the qualities of a fine midwife as she assisted me so gently in the delivery of this book. And of course all the amazing women, men and babies who have worked with me in so many different ways.

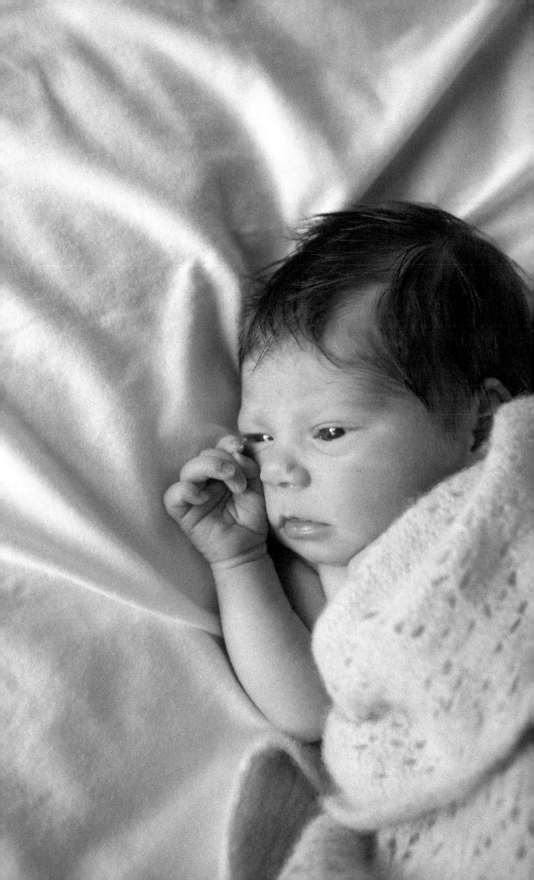

Lightning Source UK Ltd.
Milton Keynes UK
UKHW022127230419
341483UK00003B/202/P